living well with adult ADHD

Also from Russell A. Barkley

Praise for **Living Well with Adult ADHD**

"This book is a total game-changer for anyone navigating life with ADHD. Since diving in, I am already starting to build better habits and feel more in control of my life. The strategies are broken into simple, practical steps. Don't miss out!"

—Liz B., San Francisco

"This book came into my life at just the right time. The strategies aren't rigid; they're adaptable to real life, which makes them incredibly helpful. Most of all, the book is compassionate and encouraging—it helps you work with your brain, not against it. It makes ADHD feel less overwhelming and more manageable. I know I'll keep coming back to this book."

—Milo W., Richmond, Virginia

"Bravo! Drs. Knouse and Barkley have written a superb, original book. The authors have adroitly included their wealth of knowledge and experience. I love all the brief chapters in the 'Menu of Moves for Living Well' section. From 'Show Up on Time' to 'Drive Safely,' I've never seen all the major ADHD hot spots addressed so clearly, succinctly, and authoritatively."

—Edward Hallowell, MD,
coauthor of *Driven to Distraction*

"Unlike the many ADHD books that focus on neurobiology, this book gives you excellent, immediate help for dealing with common challenges. In an engaging, humorous style, Drs. Knouse and Barkley offer skillful suggestions for addressing specific issues, as well as practical strategies to improve life overall."

—Peg Dawson, EdD,
coauthor of *Smart but Scattered*

"Drs. Knouse and Barkley provide doable, bite-sized ideas that help people with ADHD figure out what they want to do and how to do it. They incorporate the latest understanding of ADHD, including the emotional impact, lifestyle factors, and how to boost self-motivation. This book is packed with everyday tactics for today's adult with ADHD."

—Margaret H. Sibley, PhD,
Department of Psychiatry and Behavioral Sciences,
University of Washington School of Medicine

THE GUILFORD LIVING WELL SERIES

The Guilford Living Well Series is designed to help individuals with common psychological conditions solve everyday problems and optimize their quality of life. Readers get specific, empathic advice for stress-proofing daily routines; navigating work, family, and relationship issues; managing symptoms effectively; and finding answers to treatment questions. Written by leading experts on each disorder, books in the series are concise, practical, and empowering.

Living Well with Bipolar Disorder
David J. Miklowitz

Living Well with OCD
Jonathan S. Abramowitz

Living Well with Psychosis
Aaron P. Brinen

Living Well with Adult ADHD
Laura E. Knouse and Russell A. Barkley

Living Well with Social Anxiety
Deborah Dobson

<u>FORTHCOMING</u>

Living Well with Depression
Christopher R. Martell

living well *with*

adult ADHD

PRACTICAL STRATEGIES
FOR IMPROVING YOUR DAILY LIFE

LAURA E. KNOUSE, PhD
RUSSELL A. BARKLEY, PhD

gp

THE GUILFORD PRESS
NEW YORK   LONDON

For B.
—L. E. K.

The information in this volume is not intended as a substitute for consultation with healthcare professionals. Each individual's health concerns should be evaluated by a qualified professional.

Printed in the United States of America

This book is printed on acid-free paper.

For product and safety concerns within the EU, please contact
GPSR@taylorandfrancis.com, Taylor & Francis Verlag GmbH, Kaufingerstraße 24, 80331 München, Germany.

Last digit is print number: 9   8   7   6   5   4   3   2   1

Library of Congress Cataloging-in-Publication Data is available from the publisher.

ISBN 978-1-4625-5512-3 (paperback) — ISBN 978-1-4625-5839-1 (hardcover)

contents

Purchasers of this book can download and print enlarged versions of select materials at *www.guilford.com/knouse-materials* for personal use or use with clients (see copyright page for details).

preface

Approximately 5.4% of adults in the United States alone have ADHD. This means that well over 14 million adults are affected by ADHD as of this writing. If you're among them, you know how impairing the disorder can be, making it difficult to function the way you want to at home and in your community, at work, and in school. This can be true even if you have received a diagnosis (many people have not) and effective treatment. You may have discovered some effective tips designed to help you get around the inattention and restlessness that are considered the hallmark symptoms of ADHD, and yet you're still dissatisfied with your quality of life.

Much advice about dealing with the challenges of ADHD is based on the idea that ADHD is strictly a disorder of inattention and hyperactivity. Having dedicated my professional life to the study of this disorder, I can say with confidence that this view is far too narrow. ADHD, I've found from years of research, is a disorder of executive functioning (EF) and the self-regulation that flows from it. We need to be able to self-regulate in all domains of life, so it's important to acquire skills and strategies that will help us compensate for the EF deficits that come with ADHD.

Enter this book. Based on her extensive knowledge and understanding of my theory of ADHD as a disorder of EF as well as of other relevant fields of psychology, Dr. Laura Knouse has compiled a toolkit overflowing with practical, effective, and even innovative methods for addressing the myriad challenges ADHD poses for responding to the demands of adult life. In the following pages you will find help with all the difficulties you encounter in your personal, occupational, and educational lives.

The skills, strategies, and other tools in the following pages also benefit from the clinical experience Dr. Knouse and I have had with evaluating and counseling hundreds of adults with ADHD as they address the many difficulties they experience. The illustrative quotes offered in the book come from clients I've worked with (either disguised to protect their privacy or composites of individuals). Before and during her writing of this text, Dr. Knouse and I discussed and even collaborated on the development and refinement of many of the tools in this book. We also pulled from other literatures—occupational, educational, and social functioning—that hold great promise for being applied to the problems of adults with ADHD.

It has therefore been both a privilege and a pleasure for me to collaborate with Dr. Knouse on this incredibly innovative and useful book for adults with ADHD. While we've consulted on the content, the writing is hers. (The *I* in the text refers to Dr. Knouse.) I have known, mentored, and worked with Dr. Knouse for 24 years, since she arrived at my clinical research lab for ADHD at the University of Massachusetts Medical Center as a student majoring in psychology at the University of Richmond. Throughout the ensuing years, she has deeply studied my theory of ADHD (and others), often using her own extensive knowledge of cognitive and behavioral psychology to derive the most useful methods for helping adults with ADHD. It's been a joy to discuss the research on ADHD, especially in adults, design research projects together, and coauthor scientific articles to share our studies of the nature and problems posed for adults with ADHD. And now this friendship and collaboration has resulted in a book that can help you live well with adult ADHD. It is an honor to have been invited to join Dr. Knouse as a coauthor of this incredibly beneficial book.

R. A. B.

acknowledgments

First and foremost, I would like to thank you, the reader, for placing unearned trust in me to pick up this book and assume you might find something valuable in its pages. Particularly if you are a person with attention-deficit/hyperactivity disorder (ADHD), I thank you for your willingness to see whether this book might have something useful to offer. In that vein, I am grateful to all the clients, research participants, friends, and family members with ADHD who have allowed me to learn from them and, in some cases, partner with them. Whatever insights this book has to offer, they are the direct result of your generosity of spirit.

I have been the beneficiary of a long list of committed mentors who have shaped my career and given me the skills and confidence to complete (nay, to even attempt!) this project. Thank you to Joan Frey Boytim, Jennifer Cable, and Jeff Riehl: When you were teaching me to sing, you were also teaching me how to write a book: how to take ownership of an endeavor through meticulous preparation, and how to trust that preparation enough to launch your work into the world, even in the presence of your doubts. Deep thanks to Catherine Bagwell for setting me on the clinical research pathway and mentoring me beyond the frame of the academic year toward my first publication.

Russ, I *literally* (as the kids say) couldn't have done it without you! From my first timid days discussing readings and running participants in your University of Massachusetts lab, you placed your confidence in me and inspired me to think more deeply, to always strive to make my work relevant to the people who need it, and to "pay it forward" by generously mentoring those whose lives I might support.

Deepest gratitude to Steve Safren for your energetic mentoring and for having enough faith in me to take me along on your ground-breaking cognitive-behavioral therapy (CBT) research adventure. Every "Good job!" still means more than you know. Sincere thanks, Susan Sprich, for your professional and personal mentoring. You are a total badass. Jen Burbridge and Bob Knauz—I can't thank you enough for your skillful supervision as I honed my CBT skills and identity as a therapist. Your confidence in me was crucial to eventually making this book a reality. So many thanks to coauthor, friend, and mentor Gill Hickman for showing me how to write a book by doing it alongside me with unshakable confidence in my ability to partner with you, the expert, in the endeavor.

It's been a great privilege to work in the smallish and collegial field of people studying psychological therapies for adults with ADHD. Shout-out to John Mitchell, my long-time friend and brilliant colleague. Although part of me thinks I'll never *really* know how old you are, I can't imagine how different (and diminished) my professional journey would have been without your friendship at the beginning. Much admiration and thanks to Russ Ramsay—your clinically grounded insights truly formed the foundation of this field, and your theoretically rich work continues to inspire. I am deeply grateful to friends and collaborators Will Canu, Cynthia Hartung, and Kate Flory—thank you for inviting me to be part of your college ADHD CBT Dream Team! I have learned so much from each of you and valued your mentoring and our deepening friendship.

The support of the University of Richmond and its passionate faculty, staff, and students have made this work possible. I am grateful for financial support of my work from the School of Arts and Sciences Faculty Research Committee as supported by the Dean's office and from the Office of the Provost. Most of all, I am thankful for the unflagging support of my faculty colleagues in the Department of Psychology for this work and the at times out-of-the-ordinary research endeavors I have pursued. Jane, Matt, Karen, Kristjen, Janelle, Arryn, Cindy, Beth, Adam, Kelly, Camilla: Your confidence has allowed me to exercise innovation in my teaching and scholarship in ways that can't be undervalued—including in my efforts to disseminate the results of my work in books like this one. I am grateful too to staff members in the University of Richmond Counseling and Psychological Services (CAPS) unit—especially Pete Leviness, Sherry Ceperich, Kris Day, and Mary Churchill, who have been willing to partner with me in creating new clinical services for students with ADHD and in supporting my research efforts. A shout-out is due to my writing accountability group partners led by the steadfast H. Bondurant—thank you for your good cheer as I plodded along toward manuscript completion. Above all, I would like to thank the many University of Richmond students who have partnered with me in learning and creating new knowledge—whether it's in the classroom, the lab (shout-out to dasLab/KNAB!), or in skills groups. Your passion to make the world a better place, despite the odds, inspires me to keep believing in that possibility and working toward it too.

Sincere thanks to Chris Benton, Kitty Moore, and The Guilford Press publishing team for putting their faith in me to create this book. Your tolerance for my out-of-the-box ideas and your patience with my excessive use of boldface and not-always-met deadlines is much appreciated, and I am so lucky that you were willing to truly partner with me in this work. Thank you! A huge thank you to Phil Hilliker for lending his design expertise in helping me figure out some of the "choose your own adventure" elements of this book. (Thanks also for running the best D&D game in town and letting me be a part of it.)

Finally, to my family—both received and chosen—thank you for laying the foundation for me to (hopefully) help others through this work. Dana, your steadfast loyalty and general bad-assery inspire me daily. Milo, your clinical insights and validation of this work helped me to pursue it. Kristin, you have always inspired me to go for it despite my overdeveloped concern about what other people think. Angie, you are the best best friend a girl could ask for, and I feel eternally lucky that someone so creative, brilliant, effective, and compassionate wants to hang out with me. Mary, thanks for putting up with being my sister! Seriously, I'm inspired by the passion you have for helping your clients, and I look forward to collaborating in the future. Mom and Dad: Thank you for unfailingly supporting my education and for bringing me up with a solid foundation of knowing I am loved *and* liked. Liam and Craig: I'm lucky to be your mom. You guys are so different from each other in ways that are delightful, but so similar in the joy you bring to others, the kindness you show, and the creative gifts you have for the world. I love you!

To Steve, my husband: You already know it all, even what I can't put into words. And these people don't get to read about it.

—L. E. K.

Enormous gratitude goes to my coauthor, Laura Knouse, for including me and my ideas in this work; to Kitty Moore of The Guilford Press for her editorial advice; Christine Benton for her extraordinary advice and editing; and the production staff at Guilford. I am also exceptionally grateful to my partner, Gabriele Meerkamper, and my sons, Steve and Ken, and their families, for their love and continued support of my work.

—R. A. B.

introduction

This book is a collection of concise, evidence-based, action-oriented steps to help you address ADHD-related challenges that get in the way of progress toward the goals that are most meaningful to you. In other words, it's a coaching manual for *living well* with ADHD.

Concise means that—despite being a professor—I'll try to communicate information efficiently and clearly. (Note that "I" throughout the book refers to Laura, the first author.)

Evidence-based means that the information and recommendations in this book are based on what we know from research about what's most helpful for adults with ADHD. The strategies in this book are also consistent with basic principles of behavior change and the way thinking influences behavior—an approach generally known as *cognitive-behavioral therapy* (CBT). So, while not every specific strategy in this book has been tested in a research study, everything recommended in this book is consistent with the emerging science of what works best for adults with ADHD.

Action-oriented means that you'll be able to make use of what you read in this book right now, today. In fact, it's the only way that anything in this book is really going to make a difference in your life. You'll try things. And then tweak the approach and try again. Then practice until that new strategy becomes the norm for you. The book is designed to help you figure out which strategies might be best to try first. I can guarantee, however, that not everything you try from this book will work for you or fit your life—but the only way to figure out what to keep and what to discard is to experiment. Even if, out of this whole book, you find only a handful of new strategies that improve your daily life, that could make a huge difference.

What Is ADHD?

I could write a book 10 times as long as this one and still not fully answer this question!* For the purpose of preparing you to use this book, it's most important for you to know the following:

• **ADHD is about problems with executive functioning— that is, how you regulate your behavior over time to meet goals.** The disorder's core symptoms can make it difficult to pursue important long-term goals over time in the face of distractions (inattention) and without responding to less important but more enticing pursuits (hyperactivity-impulsivity). The brain's tools for self-regulating are called *executive functions,* and they include self-awareness, inhibition or impulse control, working memory (remembering in order to do things), emotional self-regulation, self-motivation, and planning/problem solving. Perhaps knowing about these executive function categories can help you understand why you may struggle with meeting goals you value. They can also help you see the "why" behind many of the recommended strategies you will find throughout the book. The strategies in this book are designed to help you boost your executive functioning capacity, reduce demands on your self-regulation, or both—all in the service of pursuing what you decide is most meaningful.

• **ADHD is associated with differences in brain functioning, mostly related to genetic variation.** The executive functioning challenges experienced by people with ADHD are related to

---

*If you'd like a more comprehensive answer to this question—and, if you're new to an ADHD diagnosis, I strongly recommend it—check out *Taking Charge of Adult ADHD* by Dr. Barkley for a comprehensive and reader-friendly summary of what we know about ADHD based on the best-quality scientific research.

differences in brain functioning, and those differences are the result of *tiny variations in thousands of genes*. This means that no two people with ADHD have precisely the same disorder and symptoms, and impairment can vary tremendously from person to person. That's why it's important to recognize that not every strategy in this book will be effective or useful to you—another reason that being willing to test out different approaches is so important.

- **The impact of ADHD depends on the situation and the environment.** My guess is that you've observed this in your own life—your ADHD-related traits cause more problems in some situations than in others. Classic parent-of-kid-with-ADHD comment: "How can they have an *attention* disorder? They can pay attention to [insert name of favorite video game or other activity here] for ***hours***." Well, the truth is that some situations and tasks place more demands on executive functioning than others. The you-do-something-and-get-instant-results nature of many video games doesn't require the kind of self-regulation that, say, doing your taxes does.

The reason the situational variation of ADHD is important for our purposes is that many suggested strategies in this book are ways to "hack" the environment to reduce demands on your self-regulation. In addition, throughout the book I encourage you to reflect on ways that you can put yourself in the environments that suit you best—a strategy called *niche picking*.

- **You can learn skills to better manage the impact of ADHD on your life.** This is the single most important thing you need to know about ADHD for the purposes of this book. You are not to blame for your ADHD—you didn't choose it. But from a growing number of research studies and my firsthand experience with clients, we know that people with ADHD—including you—are capable of learning new skills and strategies that can help them get closer to the goals that are most important to them. It's probably going to be difficult. It's going to involve some false starts and some failed attempts. But everything in my experience so far tells us that, when it comes to human behavior, with the right strategies, *change is always possible*.

Is This Book for You?

It might sound egotistical, but I think this book can be for anyone who chooses to pick it up and read it. As you will see, many of the strategies provided might help anyone better manage the dizzying array of goals a person could pursue in a day, all in a world that's increasingly crowded with distractions and technology that's expertly designed to suck up all our attention. In addition, if you are a family member or friend of someone with ADHD, I hope this book can help you better understand what might be useful to your loved one.*

But most of all this book is intended to help people who find that ADHD symptoms are blocking them from doing what they want to do and being who they want to be. I've attempted to address the areas that, based on work with clients and ADHD research, seem to impact adults with ADHD the most. High school and college students with ADHD will find many of the strategies in this book useful; however, students with ADHD may also need access to strategies for studying, note taking, and other academic tasks. If you are a college student and you find the approach in this book helpful, you might benefit from my coauthored *Thriving in College with ADHD* therapist manual and student skills workbook. For a comprehensive approach for high school students, see *Parent–Teen Therapy for Executive Function Deficits and ADHD: Building Skills and Motivation* by Margaret H. Sibley.

Who I Am

I'm a clinical psychologist who has been studying ADHD and working with the adults who have it since the summer between my junior and senior years of college, when I landed a research internship in Dr. Barkley's lab at UMass medical school, where I helped him conduct a study that used a simulator to study driving in adults with ADHD. (Believe

---

*If you want to suggest any strategies from this book to a loved one with ADHD, please do so with respect for their autonomy and from a place of compassion, not nagging. You might also wish to read *When an Adult You Love Has ADHD* by Dr. Barkley.

me, we have stories.) After my experience working in Dr. Barkley's lab and completing an undergraduate honor thesis in psychology, I pursued graduate training that would allow me to continue research and clinical work with adults with ADHD. This culminated in a clinical internship and postdoctoral fellowship where I trained in the then-emerging approach of CBT for adult ADHD. I'm now professor of psychology at my alma mater, the University of Richmond, where I teach, conduct research, mentor student researchers, and collaborate with colleagues to develop and test CBT approaches for college students with ADHD. I also work with students with ADHD in our counseling center. All these experiences have shaped what I've written in this book. And I'm grateful for Dr. Barkley's collaboration on this work after many years of benefiting from his generous mentoring.

I don't have ADHD myself, so I don't know what it's like from my own direct experience. But I hope this book is authentically informed by the collaborative work I've done with people with ADHD, my former clients and students, and I hope you find it to be written in a way that is respectful and empowering. I will also note that I'm a mom of two kids, one of whom is on the autism spectrum, and that this wonderful kiddo has been receiving treatment and support since being diagnosed at age 3. While autism spectrum disorder (ASD) and ADHD are certainly different, I do think my perspective in this book—in particular, my hope that you identify what *actually matters* to you in choosing which goals to pursue—is influenced by my experience as a parent of a neurodiverse person.

Finally, I'd like to share my intentions for how I want to be toward you, the reader, as the author of this book. My aim is to be an effective coach, which means I'll strive to be:

- Encouraging—change is hard; cheerleading is necessary
- Realistic—change requires an honest assessment of where you are and what steps are reasonable
- Strategic—change requires testing out some new strategies until you find what's effective

Thanks for reading this book! I'm excited to work with you.

What This Book Is Not

- **A replacement for a comprehensive ADHD assessment by a qualified professional.** Because concentration problems can be symptoms of several mental health *and* medical disorders, ADHD can be among the most challenging conditions to diagnose accurately. No book or online quiz or primary care physician visit is a substitute for a thorough clinical evaluation that can get to the bottom of what's really going on with you and direct you toward the best toolbox of interventions. For information on finding a high-quality assessment, see the Resources at the back of the book.

- **A resource for conditions other than ADHD.** People with ADHD are at higher risk of other mental health disorders, and you may be experiencing other conditions that are affecting your functioning. While some of the strategies in this book might be useful for the problems associated with other conditions, this book is not an adequate resource for people with depression, anxiety disorders, or other conditions. Its focus is on ADHD itself.

- **A source of advice on medication for ADHD.** Medications for ADHD are an undeniably important—and sometimes life-changing—tool for managing ADHD; however, this book will focus on nonmedication strategies. (Although there will be some strategies that could help you take your medication regularly.) See the Resources at the back of the book for sources of information on medication.

- **A substitute for CBT for ADHD (or any other kind of work with a professional).** While I hope you find this book helpful, it's not a substitute for the personalized professional approach that can be provided by a well-trained cognitive-behavioral therapist. If you've found some of the strategies or the principles of this book potentially useful but need additional support to implement them in your life, seek out a professional who can provide just that. See the Resources at the back of the book for more information.

choose how to use this book

Because no two adults with ADHD have the same needs, this book is designed to be used flexibly. Read it straight through, cover to cover, if you want, but I invite you to explore some of the alternative ways you could engage. Think of this book in your hands (or on your screen) as a *Choose Your Own Adventure* book* for learning more about yourself and how to live well with ADHD.

There are three major sections in the rest of the book:

- **Part One, the Toolbox:** Provides coaching in a range of tried-and-true skills that have helped many people live well with adult ADHD.

- **Part Two, the Menu:** Breaks down specific challenges you may experience as an adult with ADHD and directs you to possible skills and solutions (including tools for the Toolbox). Most chapters in the Menu begin with some questions you'll answer to zero in on your specific needs.

- **Part Three, the Principles:** Invites you to reflect on what living well means to you and lays out the Principles underlying the recommendations in this book. You can use the Principles to help you

---

*Yes, I grew up in the 1980s.

adapt the tools or invent new ones, to help you remember to use strategies at key moments, or to replenish your motivation when needed.

> **Important:** You will notice that there is a lot of cross-referencing in the book—places where I refer you to other pages or sections. This is because lots of the ideas and skills connect to one another, and I didn't want to repeat too much. To help you navigate, as you read you may want to have nearby:
>
> - Sticky notes, paper clips, or bookmarks
> - A notebook where you will jot down your ideas as you engage with the book (I've provided blanks for you to jot down replies to prompts throughout the book; you can either do that right in the book or use your notebook.)

Three Pathways

While you can jump into the book anywhere you like, here are three pathways you could take based on your needs. Read the descriptions and then mark off which pathway fits your needs best.

- **The Nuts-and-Bolts Pathway:** For readers who are eager to build foundational skills or readers who have developed some coping skills and are interested in new techniques they haven't mastered yet. You will start with picking up skills from the Toolbox, followed by examples of ways to apply those tools in the Menu, and finally see how these examples play out in terms of big-picture principles for living.

- **The Targeted Pathway:** For readers who have a clear idea of their biggest needs and want some possible solutions as soon as possible, the targeted pathway is the way to go. Choose sections from the Menu that meet your needs and you'll be directed to specific skills from the Toolbox that can help. Later you might benefit from going deeper with the Principles section.

- **The Big-Picture Pathway:** For readers who like to start with the Big Ideas and then learn more about the specifics. Choose this pathway if you like to start by reflecting on your own goals and motivations. You'll start with the Principles, then learn about how they show up in the skills in the Toolbox, followed by application to specific problems in the Menu.

Mark the pathway in the diagram below that suits you best.

These are only suggestions—the best pathway through the book is one that will keep you reading and, most importantly, trying out these skills and ideas in your real life. So explore, engage, and see what works!

☐ **The Nuts-and-Bolts Pathway**

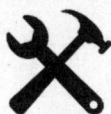   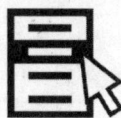   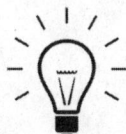

Toolbox   Menu   Principles

☐ **The Targeted Pathway**

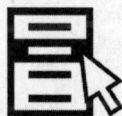   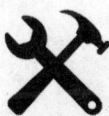   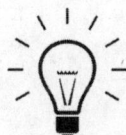

Menu   Toolbox   Principles

☐ **The Big-Picture Pathway**

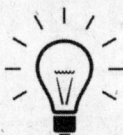   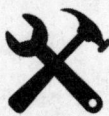   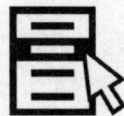

Principles   Toolbox   Menu

PART ONE

your ADHD toolbox

If anyone tells you there's a one-size-fits-all solution to the problems that ADHD causes in life, be *very* skeptical. Each person, each situation, each moment is different. Managing ADHD (and life in general) involves flexibly applying tools and strategies to figure out "what works" in each situation you find yourself in.

Responding flexibly demands a variety of tools in your metaphorical ADHD Toolbox. You might visualize a traditional set of home repair tools, but if that's not interesting to you, choose a tool set that's more personally meaningful, such as:

- Your drawer of kitchen tools
- Your car detailing kit
- Your collection of art supplies
- Your package of editing programs, settings, and filters
- Your gardening tools
- Your knitting or sewing tools and supplies
- Your idea here: _____

Whatever you choose, recognize that you need enough tools to do a variety of jobs and the ability to switch tools if needed. This is exactly how you should think of your ADHD Toolbox.

It's also important to recognize that putting a new tool in your box is only the first step. Like learning to use any new tool, it will take time and practice. And sometimes that will be hard, and you'll feel like you're not making progress, and you might want to give up. And when it gets hard, remember this:

No one thing always works.

If something isn't working, it doesn't mean that you'll never figure it out or that the tool you chose is worthless. It means that life is a moving target, and you may have to try again, choose a different tool, show yourself kindness—and sometimes do all three. That's just how it goes.

But sometimes things *will* work. And sometimes you'll get a little bit better at recognizing what to try next time. And over time, bit by bit, you will find you're living better and better with your ADHD.

Tools for the Toolbox

In this book *tools* include any device, skill, or strategy you can use to change your behavior, mood, thoughts, or environment in a way that could help you live in the direction of your goals. Throughout the Menu section of the book, I'll refer back to these tools when one applies to a particular problem. And I hope that you'll find uses for these tools that I haven't thought of.

As you try out the tools in this section, add your favorites to your Tools and Strategies Log (available to download and print at *www. guilford.com/knouse-materials*). You can also use a notebook, electronic document, or notes app to record your progress and ideas.

But **please** keep in mind:

> You don't have to use *all* the tools!

Otherwise, this Toolbox could easily feel overwhelming. No one expects you to add *all* these tools to your box. That's not the goal. The goal is to develop a collection of tools that works for you and *your* needs—not to meet someone else's expectations. Finding even one new, effective tool that you use consistently could change your life for the better. (Believe me; I've seen it happen.)

Yeah, Right—I've Tried a Bunch of These Before

That's probably true. Nevertheless, as you look through the Toolbox, please keep an open mind. You may have tried using some of these tools, but they didn't work as well as you'd hoped. Maybe you're having thoughts like "I've tried to use a planner a million times, and it just doesn't work for me" or "I'm just a disorganized person, and no tool is going to change all that."

There might be least some truth to thoughts like these. It's your brain's way of using your past experience to help you predict the future. But those predictions might also be wrong. They might block you from discovering a way that a tool really *could* work for you. So consider the possibility that what hasn't worked just hasn't worked *yet*.

To discover what works for you, for each new tool, you will need to:

> **Commit to a warm-up phase.**

It's important to give yourself and the tool a chance to get used to each other. Any new skill, new relationship, new anything may feel clunky at first, so it's important not to quit at the first sign of awkwardness. Give the tool time to feel comfortable in your hands. I recommend *at least a week of tryout* for each tool, adjusting as you go. This won't be easy, but it might be worth it—there's only one way to find out.

1

tools for organizing time and tasks

Adulting requires managing appointments, tasks, and deadlines. Tools that tell you **what** to do **when** are crucial. Maybe when you were younger—when your brain was quicker and you had fewer things to manage—you could hold everything you needed to do in your mind without using any tools. But for most adults that's an unreasonable expectation—especially if you're an adult with ADHD.

Most of us need add-ons to our memory and planning capacity—like mental wheelbarrows that let you carry five times as many heavy objects as you could using just your arms. The tools in this chapter are designed to enhance your brain power by allowing you to offload information and visualize it in a way that will help you decide **what** to do **when**. Lots of other tools and strategies in this book rely on the tools in this chapter—so consider these foundational tools in your box.

You may have tried tools like this before and struggled. That's okay and not unexpected. It's true that, for people with ADHD, it can be harder to make these tools into habits. But from years of working with adults with ADHD, I've seen time and again that people with ADHD can learn to use these strategies and improve their lives. It might just take a little more time, repetition, or tweaking. The idea is to practice using the tool until it feels strange *not* to use it.

Calendar System

A Calendar System is an absolute essential in any adult ADHD Toolbox. This tool tells you what's coming up and how long you have to prepare for it, reducing unpleasant surprises in your life.

Your Calendar System can be on paper, or it can be digital. There are pros and cons to each. I will admit that I am a huge Google Calendar fan because of its visual layout and the ability to link information to each appointment, set reminders, and access the calendar on my phone or computer. But some people are die-hard paper planner devotees. What's best is what works for you.

Importantly, you should choose the system that will allow you to follow the calendar rules shown on the facing page. These rules are designed to help you make the most of the calendar and fast-track your way to making it a habit.

Will you use a paper calendar or a digital calendar? If digital, which one?

I'll try using: _____

_____

Will your choice help you stick to the calendar rules? **yes no**

(If no, choose a different system.)

Great! Now that you've chosen the tool you want to build into a habit, it's time to commit to the calendar practice rule.

You have to test-drive your Calendar System, committing to the calendar rules shown on the facing page *for at least a week* before deciding to switch to a different system.

Why? Any new tool will feel clunky at first. People with ADHD tend to really like novel things, so in the early stages of learning anything new, it can be tempting to switch to a new, brighter, shinier tool. The problem is that frequent switching means you won't spend enough time with a system to make it an automatic habit.

Calendar rules	But why?
Use only one Calendar System for yourself.	Using more than one system means different information can end up in different places. Confusing!
You need access to the calendar at all times.	You need to be able to add to your calendar and check it anytime, anywhere.
Put all appointments and schedule items in the calendar right away.	The calendar is useful only if it's an accurate reflection of your life.
Check your calendar several times per day.	The calendar is useful only if you're . . . using it.

Task-Tracking System

Some form of the classic "to-do" list is an utter necessity in any ADHD Toolbox. This tool gives you a comprehensive view of everything that's on your plate so that you can distribute your time and effort strategically—that is, prioritize. (More about this in the next section.)

Your Task-Tracking System can be on paper—such as a section in your planner or just a notepad—or it can be digital, and there are pluses and minuses to each. Task-tracker apps can contain a huge range of features, but really all you need is the ability to add items to a list, label or sort them in some way, and check them off. (So satisfying!) My personal favorite app for personal task tracking is Trello. I've had lots of clients say they like Google Keep.

Whatever you choose, pick a system that will allow you to best follow the task-tracker rules shown on the next page. Like the calendar rules, these rules are designed to help you fast-track your way to a task list habit.

Will you use a paper or a digital task tracker? If digital, which one?

I'll try using: _____

_____

Task-tracker rules	But why?
Use only one task tracker for yourself. (No notes on scraps of paper or sticky notes everywhere!)*	Using more than one system means different information can end up in different places. Confusing!
You need access to the Task-Tracking System at all times.	You need to be able to add to your task tracker and check it anytime, anywhere.
Put all to-do tasks into the tracker right away.	Tasks not in the tracker will get missed.
Check your task tracker several times per day.	The tracker is useful only if you're . . . using it.

*Sticky notes are *excellent* tools for placing reminders in strategic locations—just don't use them as your method for overall task tracking.

Will your choice help you stick to the task-tracker rules?
yes   no

(If no, choose a different system.)

Great! Now that you've chosen the tool you want to build into a habit, it's time to commit to that important practice rule: using the system *for at least a week* before trying something else.

Priority Labeling (or Sorting)

Looking at a giant list of to-be-done tasks can be intimidating because **everything** can feel urgent. To deploy your time and effort efficiently, you'll need to add a Priority Labeling (or Sorting) system to your Task-Tracking System. Then you'll have a better idea of where to focus your attention and effort.

Follow these steps:

1. Label each task in your tracker with a **due date** based on information from your Calendar System.

2. For tasks without a definite due date, label these with **the date by which you'd like to complete the task**—*your* due date.

3. Next, label each task based on how important you think it is. In other words, how big a difference it will ultimately make in your life if you do (or don't) get it done. Try your best to give this rating without paying attention to how urgent the task is (that is, the due date).

4. Finally, use the due dates and the importance rating to label or sort each task into priority categories. Adapting work by Dr. Steven Safren, I recommend the following categories:

A Tasks: Very urgent and important. They need to be done today or tomorrow.

B Tasks: Not as urgent, but still important. Some part needs to get done in the next few days. Break off part of a B task and make that an A task.

C Tasks: Not really urgent or important but may be easy. Be careful not to get stuck doing just these!

By *label or sort* I mean you can literally write *A, B,* or *C* next to the task, color-code it, or create separate lists for each priority rating. For example, using Trello, I can put each task on a little virtual card with its own due date and then create columns or stacks of these cards. Using Trello, you could create your "A Stack" on the far left followed by your "B Stack" and "C Stack" to the right across the screen.* Then just drag and drop the task items as they change in priority over time.

This seems really tedious. Am I going to have to do this for every task? Forever?

Well, sort of. Like any of the tools, Priority Labeling (or Sorting) is going to feel clunky at first, but with practice, applying these labels will become second nature.

Now the hard part . . .

---

*In reality I have my stacks labeled according to when I need to work on and complete the task: "Today's Tasks" on the far left, followed by "This Week's Tasks," followed by "Future Tasks." But now I'm thinking I should try A, B, C instead! Also important: Do I always stick to completing everything on my daily list or doing the tasks in the "correct" priority order? Answer: Absolutely not, *but* using this priority system helps me complete a larger number of important tasks than I would if I just did tasks willy-nilly.

The bottom line: *Doing the system perfectly isn't the point.* The point is to make your use of the system good enough to produce some benefit.

Now that you know your priorities, you need to devote your time and effort to A tasks *before* B tasks *before* C tasks. It sounds simple, but it's actually pretty difficult because more important tasks usually have a lot of steps, so they can't give you the satisfaction of immediate completion. You might look at an A or B task and just feel gross or overwhelmed—like you want to do **anything** else.

This is how we get stuck in C-task land, checking our email or tidying our desk when we know we should be doing something more urgent or important. Some people call this "productive procrastination" or "procrastivity," but unfortunately it's often quite unproductive and can create stress in your life.

Fortunately, there are other tools that you can use to help you bring your efforts in line with your priorities. The next chapter describes these tools.

2

tools for starting, stopping, and finishing

Knowing *what* to do *when* is only the first half of the equation when it comes to getting your actions to line up with your intentions and goals. A lot of the time the hardest part is simply *doing* the thing. And adults with ADHD often report having difficulties getting started on important things, even when they *know* what's important.

What's sometimes less obvious is that problems *getting started* can be the result of difficulty *stopping* doing other things. Although there's not much solid scientific research on it yet, many adults with ADHD report difficulties controlling "hyperfocus" states—that is, getting so wrapped up in a rewarding task or activity that they lose awareness of time and of other tasks that might need their attention. Shifting your attention—or task switching—might be difficult for you without some extra tools in that Toolbox. In the Menu section, I specifically address hyperfocus in Chapters 4 and 11. For now, let's put the tools in the Toolbox that can help you manage it.

Clocks, Watches, and Timers

Timekeeping devices can be powerful tools to help people—with and without ADHD—shift tasks when they need to. Consider integrating more of these devices into your environment and into your daily life and using them in the following ways.

Clocks

Placing more clocks in your environment can improve your awareness of time, which can be particularly important for adults with ADHD who have less accurate "internal clocks" to perceive the passage of the hours. Fortunately, there are lots of attractive options if you want to add more clocks to your life. (Classic Kit-Cat Klock, anyone?) Location is important here. For example, does it seem like you fall into a time warp when doing your morning bathroom routine? Put a clock there.

Watches

Watches have the added advantage of following you around everywhere you go. Sure your mobile phone has a clock you can check, but a watch is attached to your body in a way that makes it maximally accessible. In addition, watches can be programmed with alarms, and those that sync with your phone can deliver vibrating alarms and reminders synced with your Calendar System.

Timers

Timers have been an especially powerful and flexible tool for many of the adults with ADHD that I've worked with. They come in many forms from timer apps on your phone to the timers on your oven or microwave to stand-alone models from an old-school hourglass to plastic cubes that time different durations depending on which side you put them on (my personal favorite).

Timers are useful for **both** starting and stopping. For starting, if there's a task you can't stand and you're having trouble getting started, it might be easier to commit to *just 10 minutes* of that task. You only have to commit do doing the task until the timer rings. And you might find that once you get started, it's not so bad.

For stopping tasks that suck you in, you can set a timer before you begin the task and use the alarm as a signal to stop. If you want to get even fancier, there are integrated timers for apps and web browsers that can shut off access to certain activities when a certain amount of use time is up. For more information on these, see Switch Gears When You Need To (Chapter 11), Section A (page 104).

Alarms, Reminders, and Prompts

Many of the tasks you do in a day must be done in a certain location or at a certain time. You need to take your medication in the bathroom each morning before you leave the house. You have to put the garbage out by the road every other Thursday evening. You have to grab your gym bag before going out the door in the morning on days that you have after-work volleyball practice. It's a lot to manage!

If you have ADHD, it may be difficult to remember when and where to do things throughout your complex day. Alarms, Reminders, and Prompts can help take the load off your brain and instead put the work of remembering into the environment around you.

Check out the table on the next page for examples of these tools and consider how you can use them in your daily life.

You can get really creative with these methods of "hacking the environment." Here's one of my favorite suggestions from a former student with ADHD.

This student would often buy lots of healthy fruits and vegetables but then forget about them in the crisper drawer until they were spoiled and had to be thrown away. She hacked the refrigerator environment by swapping the produce in the crisper drawers with the condiments on the door shelves. That way, the fruits and veggies were literally "in her

Alarms, Reminders, and Prompts

	Alarm	Reminder	Prompt
What is it?	A *signal* (usually a sound) that it's time to do something	A *statement* of what you need to do at a particular place or occasion	An *object* in your environment that nudges you toward an action
When is it useful?	When you need to do something at a specific time or by a deadline	When you need to do something (or not do something!) at a particular location or at a time that you're typically in that location	When you need to do something at a particular location and use an object or item to do it
Examples	• Add an alarm to an appointment in your online calendar to go off at the time you need to leave the house (or before) • Set an alarm that also darkens your phone screen when it's time to go to bed	• Put a sticky note on your bathroom mirror: "Is it Thursday? Did you put the trash out?" • Record a voice memo of the items you need to get at the store and link it to that task in your calendar	• Hang your gym bag on the doorknob of the front door • Duct-tape your medication bottle to your toothbrush

Note: The difference between these three tools is really subtle and not super important, but I've separated them out to encourage you to think of new, creative ways to use tools like this in your daily life.

face" every time she opened the fridge, while the condiments—which keep for a long time and have specific uses—were tucked away but ready when she needed to go looking for them. And now this is what my fridge looks like too.

This is a great example of creating *prompts* for desired behavior, but it's just one example of how you can hack your environment. Be creative, have fun—and let me know what you come up with!

Reduced-Distraction Environments

One of the most important ways you can hack your environment when you have ADHD is to engineer a personalized setup for maximizing your focus and minimizing distractions when you need to do deep work. If you struggle with ADHD, your threshold for getting distracted may be lower than other people's—especially when you're working on a task that's boring or anxiety provoking. This section will help you engineer a personalized environment that will reduce the temptation to divert your attention elsewhere.

Step 1: Do a Distraction Inventory

The best way to do this is to *actually sit down and try to work on a boring task.* When you get distracted (because you will), use the chart on page 26 to make a note of the causes of that distraction (another copy is available for downloading and printing at *www.guilford.com/knouse-materials*).

Step 2: Plan Your Reduced-Distraction Environments

Based on what you observed in Step 1, map out ways to prevent or manage the distractions that get you off track. I've provided you with some ideas that have worked for my clients to get started.

- **Ideas for managing sound:** Earplugs or earmuffs, noise-canceling headphones, focus-friendly playlists on a streaming service (there's a whole Focus category on Spotify), recordings of ambient sounds like rain, white noise, or coffee shop sounds; actually working in a coffee shop.
- **Ideas for managing visuals:** Working in a private space, switching up the lighting, adding pleasant visuals like plants, curtains, or blinds to adjust lighting.
- **Ideas for managing tech:** Turning off text or email notifications on devices, turning your phone off before working, putting your phone away in your bag or in a drawer, using apps like Freedom,

CAUSES OF DISTRACTION

Source of distraction	Examples	Notes
Sounds	Noises in the room, silence, people talking in the background	
Sights	Fluorescent lights, pets or kids moving around	
Tech	Phone buzzing, email notifications, pop-up ads, checking certain websites	
Thoughts and feelings	Anxious thoughts, thoughts about other things you should be doing, feeling restless	
Other		

BlockSite, or StayFocusd to restrict your access to certain sites while working.

• **Ideas for managing thoughts and feelings:** Writing down your distracting thoughts on a notepad while working to deal with them later; using the Pomodoro Technique (page 32) to build in structured breaks; using a fidget toy, standing desk, or other type of physical movement to manage internal restlessness.

You can jot down your answers to the following questions in the blanks or in your notebook.

Environment 1: Where will you work, and what strategies will you have in place to reduce distractions?

Where? _____

What strategies?

1. _____

2. _____

3. _____

Environment 2: Where will you work, and what strategies will you have in place to reduce distractions?

Where? _____

What strategies?

1. _____

2. _____

3. _____

Step 3: Set It Up + Reminders

Now use your plan to set up your Reduced-Distraction Environments or get what you need to act on your strategies.

Important: How will you remember to actually use these strategies when you need them?

I recommend that you *create reminders of your Reduced-Distraction Environments plan,* so you can remember what you need to be most successful. You could:

- Write your plan on a sticky note that goes inside your planner or on your laptop cover
- Make a sign to post in your desk area
- Write your plan on a virtual sticky note that's on your computer desktop

Task Chunks

The most important and meaningful tasks in your life are often the ones that are most complicated. Many important tasks are really a long chain of individual tasks knitted together to make a series of hurdles you have to tackle one at a time. Take for example income taxes. If you do them yourself, you need to assemble all your paperwork and then follow a long series of tedious steps before you can hit "submit."

Imagine you've added "Do taxes" to your task tracker. How do you think you'll feel when you look at that task? Probably *not* "Yessss! I can't WAIT to do this task!" It's probably the opposite, something like "Ugh, I don't have time to do that now" or "That feels too overwhelming; I can do it later." In an instance like this, you need to break off Task Chunks that are *very specific* and *more reasonable* to tackle.

For "Do taxes," the Task Chunks might be:

1. Make an account on OnlineTaxes.com*
2. Use the website to make a list of needed documents
3. Gather needed documents to a folder (electronic or paper)

---

*Not a real site, but just go with me on this.

4. Start your online return

5. Tackle one section of the tax return and hit "save"

6. Continue until you can submit

How do Task Chunks help you accomplish things? Let's do an experiment—look at these two list items and compare how you'd feel if given a choice between them:

Choice 1: Do taxes.

Choice 2: Make an account on OnlineTaxes.com.

Which one feels ickier? More vague? And which one are you more likely to avoid?

If you're like me, you'd probably be more likely to tackle Choice 2 because it tells you exactly what do to, it doesn't seem like it would take forever, and you'll be able to check it off your list quickly. And once you make that account on the tax site, it's possible you'll go ahead to the next step anyway—an example of what psychologists call *behavioral momentum.*

So, if you look at a task on your list and feel the urge to avoid it ("Ugh!"), it's time to break that task into chunks, add those chunks to your task list, and tackle the first chunk.

Rewarding Consequences

When it comes to motivation problems, the absolute worst advice I can think of is the classic Nike tagline: "Just do it." Why? Because trying to force yourself to do something rarely works in the absence of other motivators. One of the most powerful motivators is the *immediate consequence of an action*—that is, what comes directly after the behavior. If an action has been followed by Rewarding Consequences in the past, it's more likely to happen again. And if you know you'll be able to access a reward right after an action, that reward can help to pull your behavior along toward the goal.

You pick up your phone; you can check the latest news. You open the refrigerator; you can see an array of rewarding foods. You turn on the shower; warm water flows over you. Every tiny action you do in a day is pulled along by its immediate consequences.

You can harness the power of Rewarding Consequences and use them to help you get started on tasks and see them through to completion. Rewarding Consequences can include:

- Access to a rewarding item, like a cup of coffee
- Access to enjoyable activities, like watching a favorite video on YouTube*
- Praise or positive attention from someone you respect
- Escape from a hard task by taking a short break

To use Rewarding Consequences most powerfully, consequences must be:

• **Clearly stated:** Write down your reward plan by using "If I do [specific task description], then I can [rewarding consequence]" as a model. An example would be "If I spend 30 minutes doing the dishes, then I can watch an episode of *Parks and Recreation*."

• **Immediate:** Choose Rewarding Consequences you can access right away.

• **Meaningful:** Be sure it's something you actually value enough to be motivated by.

• **Right-sized:** At the same time, make sure the Rewarding Consequences aren't too big or time-consuming in proportion to the task. When in doubt, break tasks into small pieces and follow them with small rewards versus expecting yourself to do a massive task for an equally massive reward.

---

*Oddly, rewarding activities don't have to be enjoyable. Any activity that's more preferred than the activity you're trying to reward can work as a motivator. You could reward yourself with the opportunity to do an easier chore if you do a harder chore beforehand—in other words, "do the worst first."

Among the most important ideas behind these strategies is that the rewards for doing a task must be greater than those positive consequences for not doing it. Or its corollary, the reasons for not doing a task must be far more aversive than those involved in getting it done. Either way there must be a sizable imbalance in these incentives to motivate you to start the task. So arranging the consequences of doing and not doing a task is a critical part of getting work done.

Let's try this out. Pick a task from your Task-Tracking System (page 17) that should take about 30 minutes and then think of a Rewarding Consequence that seems right-sized for that task.

If I _____ *then* I will _____

Now either test out this action-consequence immediately *or* put it in your Calendar System to try later today. Continue to look for ways to work Rewarding Consequences into your daily life by following less preferred activities with more preferred, rewarding activities.

Strategic Task Scheduling

Another way to help you get started on important but avoided tasks is to make a specific and strategic appointment with yourself. Here you'll use your Calendar System and the power of Rewarding Consequences to increase the likelihood that you'll get started on something you've been putting off.

To schedule strategically, follow these steps:

1. Choose a task that you have been avoiding.
2. Break off a chunk that will last no more than 30–60 minutes.
3. Choose a time on your calendar to schedule the task. Consider an optimal time of day for you.
4. Schedule the task in the slot you chose.
5. Schedule a Rewarding Consequence right afterward. Literally write the consequence in the calendar.

For the Rewarding Consequence, you might leverage rewarding things that naturally happen throughout your day, such as an already-scheduled lunch with a friend, and schedule the avoided task right beforehand.

Another version of Strategic Task Scheduling is *temptation bundling*. You can use this strategy when an avoided task *can be done simultaneously* with a rewarding task. For example:

- Watching your favorite show while running on the treadmill
- Listening to a beloved podcast while washing the dishes
- Listening to the new Taylor Swift album while folding the laundry
- Turning on your essential oil diffuser while doing your taxes
- Drinking your favorite tea while grading papers

Importantly, temptation bundling works best if you **only** *let yourself do the rewarding thing when you're doing the avoided task* and at no other times. This can sometimes be a problem for people when no one else knows of this private contract you have made with yourself. The opportunity to cheat the agreement with yourself is always present. To undercut this temptation, it is often recommended that you disclose your contract with yourself to someone else with whom you are friendly, when possible, as such public accountability for self-change can go a long way toward ensuring that the agreement is fulfilled.

The Pomodoro Technique

When you have a lengthy, unexciting task that you just can't seem to start or sustain, it's time to break out the big guns: the Pomodoro Technique. It was invented by Francesco Cirillo when, as a university student, he needed to buckle down and get a lot of studying done. Here it's adapted to help you manage ADHD-related distractibility and motivation challenges.

The classic Pomodoro method uses these steps (but read on to see how to make them more user-friendly for a person with ADHD):

1. Write down the Task Chunk you need to work on.

2. Set a timer for 25 minutes (25 minutes = 1 Pomodoro).

3. Work on the task until time is up.

4. Take a 5-minute break.

5. Every 4 Pomodoros, take a longer break (20–30 minutes).

> **Important:** Many adults with ADHD find that they need to work up to being able to focus for longer periods of time. So start with a smaller work period, like 5 minutes, and follow that with a very short break—like 2 minutes—then repeat. Your goal is to eventually increase the timer duration to 25 minutes but not make the breaks so long that you get distracted by finding something more interesting to do. And for some people, 25 minutes will always be too long. Adults with ADHD typically say that their sweet spot for Pomodoro work periods is somewhere between 8 and 20–25 minutes. Whatever the interval that leads to success at sustained work, that is the Pomodoro interval for you.

I'd describe Pomodoro as a mega-tool because it combines three of our Starting and Stopping tools into one: a timer,* Task Chunks, and Rewarding Consequences (that is, the 5-minute break). And fortunately there are lots of apps based on Pomodoro that you can use to structure your work time. Search for one in the app store, choose a task from your task tracker, and give this tool a test drive.

Accountability Partners

For most humans, approval and support from others are powerful rewards that can motivate our behavior when the task-related going gets tough. Accountability Partners are people who have committed to helping you stay on track toward your goals.

---

*The technique is named for the tomato-shaped kitchen timer Cirillo used (*pomodoro* is Italian for tomato).

Accountability partnerships may:

- Be a one way street—like coaching—or based on partners offering mutual support
- Be pair or group based, such as an accountability group
- Be one shot or ongoing
- Range from minimal interaction and support—like simply working in the same space as another person—to higher degrees of feedback and support

Body doubling is a popular minimal interaction version of accountability partnership. Partners simply work alongside each other in a physical or virtual space, and their mutual presence helps them stay focused and on task. For those wishing to stick to an exercise routine, scheduling runs or gym visits with a workout buddy can help you stick to your intentions.*

For people trying to tackle long-term solitary projects, such as writing a book, *accountability groups* offer a space for mutual motivation and empathy. For example, I wrote this book with the support of a Summer Writing Accountability Group at the University of Richmond.** We met for 1 hour per week to body double while writing and used a shared Google Doc to set our weekly and daily goals, to track our progress, and to use comments and emojis to provide encouragement and feedback to each other.

The most important step in a successful accountability partnership (and most relationships!) is setting clear expectations. If you're considering setting up a partnership, use the prompts that follow to plan your ask.

What is the task you want to accomplish or the behavior you want to sustain?

_____

---

*I stumbled on the ultimate version of the workout accountability partnership—I'm the instructor for my fitness classes (Jazzercise!), so I really *must* show up.

**Shout out to H., Lauren, Abigail, and Jannette!

What type of support do you think you need? (Check all that apply.)

- ❑ Presence of another person (body doubling; workout buddy)
- ❑ Praise or positive affirmation
- ❑ Empathy with struggles
- ❑ Feedback or suggestions for improvement
- ❑ Administering Rewarding Consequences (other than praise)

Would you prefer:

- ❑ A one-way partnership (coaching)
- ❑ A two-way partnership (mutual accountability)
- ❑ A group

Who in your life might be able to provide this type of support?*
(If you're not sure, write down some ideas for how to identify people who could be good partners—for example, online affinity groups, others at your gym, and so on.)

_____

Decide with your Accountability Partner(s):

How frequently will you meet or check in? (It should be at least weekly.)

_____

How long will this partnership last?

_____

*Exercise caution if you're considering your spouse or intimate partner as an Accountability Partner. Even the healthiest of these relationships have complicated dynamics that might make an accountability partnership more messy than helpful.

Where will you meet (physical or virtual)?

_____

What will you do during meetings or check-ins?

_____

Choice Point Analysis

When it comes to starting and stopping tasks, it pays to attend to what's going on inside your body and mind. At hundreds of *choice points* throughout the day, we experience feelings and thoughts that mark or influence which actions we choose. Becoming aware of your inner world can be an important tool toward making more intentional choices about what to do in a given moment.

Here are some examples. As you read them, *underline or highlight* anything that feels familiar to you.

You really want to commit to a regular exercise routine, so you can feel better and lower the risk of heart disease, which runs in your family. You set the goal of working out on 4 of the 7 days in the upcoming week. But now it's Day 5, and you haven't even worked out once. You feel ashamed and angry at yourself. You think, "Just another example of how I've failed again. Why can't I be a real adult and control myself? It's ruined now." You start playing on your phone to distract yourself from feeling bad and don't go to the gym today or any other day the rest of the week.

It's 9:00 P.M., and you haven't done the dishes yet, even though you promised your partner you'd do that chore daily this week. (A clean kitchen is really important to helping you and your partner feel less stressed out.) You're lying on the couch watching Netflix, and the next episode of your show starts automatically. You think about getting up to wash the dishes and feel a sense of exhaustion. You think to yourself, "I can watch just one more episode and then do those dishes. I worked hard today and deserve it." You fall asleep on the couch and wake up at 2:00 A.M.

You've got a big presentation for work due on Friday, and it's late on Tuesday. You have another hour left before you have to leave to pick up your child at day care. You look at "work on presentation" on your task tracker and feel a sense of disgust ("Ugh!"). You think to yourself, "I don't have enough time to really get started on this now anyway—I have plenty of time tomorrow. I work better under pressure anyway." You spend the hour working on an easy task that's not due for another month.

What did you notice from the examples above? Did anything feel familiar? If so, what?

_____

_____

_____

Here are a few more things to notice about these examples:

1. Each scenario has a *choice point* where an important but more difficult task takes a back seat to something less important. These situations are very common in the everyday lives of adults whether they have ADHD or not, but adults with ADHD may experience them even more often.

2. The effects of moments like these add up. It's not a terrible or wrong thing when a person decides to put off a task until later. There can be really good reasons for doing so, and I'm not saying it's good for people to be working, working, working continuously. (To be clear, that is not healthy.) But spending the *majority* of your time putting off important tasks can lead to increased stress, relationship or employment problems, and the sense that you're not accomplishing important goals in your life.

3. Each choice point is accompanied by feelings and thoughts that mark or influence the decision to put off the important task. Although not every choice has feelings and thoughts you can notice, when you look back on your experiences, you might be able to identify signals like these.

Becoming aware of your own patterns of feelings and thoughts at task choice points can take some practice, so there's a specific tool you can use to get better at it: the Choice Point Analysis. Choice Point Analysis forms are available to download and print at *www.guilford.com/ knouse-materials*.

1. Choose a recent time when you put off an important task and it later caused problems for you. What was the task?

    _____

2. Why was this task important to you?

    _____

3. When you made the choice, where were you? What was going on?

    _____

4. When you thought about the important task in that moment, how did you feel?

    _____

5. What thoughts went through your head?

    _____

6. What did you do *instead of* the important task?

    _____

7. Do any of your answers seem *old*? Like maybe they've happened a lot before? These are things to look out for in the future.

    _____

Congrats! You've completed your first Choice Point Analysis. Whenever you realize you've put off doing a task or made some other choice that didn't serve you in the long run, stop and ask yourself these questions. Even if you realize it later, do the Choice Point Analysis for practice.

As mentioned, you can find blank Choice Point Analysis forms—one for choices in general and one for procrastination—to download and print at *www.guilford.com/knouse-materials*. Over time you may begin to notice that particular situations, thoughts, and feelings signal that you're about to avoid a task.

It may seem strange, but *the goal of the Choice Point Analysis isn't to change anything*—rather, the goal is to gather some clues about what might be going on so that you can become more aware and have a fighting chance of "catching yourself" and making a different decision in the future.

Awareness is the first step.

But it takes time and practice! One idea for improving your awareness of choice points is to take note of the thoughts that come up for you frequently in these moments. I sometimes refer to these frequent but frequently problematic thoughts as personal *red flag thoughts*. When you notice them coming up, you may be in a moment where alternative strategies are needed. For example, you might "know" you need to leave for an appointment but have thoughts like "I just need to finish this one thing first" or "Just 5 more minutes . . . " and end up delaying departure until you've made yourself late and stressed out. Reread the scenarios on page 36 and see if you can identify the red flag thoughts in them.

Can you identify any personal *red flag thoughts* from the Choice Point Analysis you completed above? If so, write them here:

_____

_____

_____

How can you become more aware of these thoughts? You could create reminders (page 24). For example, one of my former clients wrote his most tenacious red flag thought on a sticky note and put it in his workspace—the spot where he experienced that thought most frequently. Or you could add helpful coaching statements to the appointment reminder that pops up on your phone—maybe something like "It's almost time to leave! Be nice to the You of the Future and give her enough time." (It's goofy, but it just might work.)

Once you've gotten some practice with the Choice Point Analysis, check out the final mega-skill for starting and stopping . . .

Self-Coaching

If you can start noticing when you're at a choice point, you can start to use Self-Coaching: a key strategy for increasing the chances that you'll be able to make better choices—at least some of the time. And remember—this isn't about perfection. Even a few more times of making a better choice can add up to a huge difference over time. And with practice you'll be able to successfully use Self-Coaching more and more often.

I'm using coaching as a metaphor here on purpose. I really want you to think about how you can be your own most effective coach and self-motivator. This is your life, and the stakes are high! How do you want to show up for yourself in these tough choice point moments?

How about:

"You've already messed up bad, so why should you even bother?"

"It's never going to work anyway—this is how you are."

"It's no big deal. You don't really need to use any of these tools. It's all gonna work out in the end."

"You'll *definitely* feel like tackling that hard thing tomorrow. Just take a break!"

What do you think? Do these seem like the kinds of things an effective coach would say to their players? Would you feel good about a coach who said these things to your child or someone else you care about?

Yet *this is how we talk to ourselves* in tough choice point moments! There must be a better way . . .

In my experience, better coaching is a matter of being strategic and supportive:

- **Strategic** coaching actually tells you what you can do to improve. It's not just a generic ***"Do it!"***

- **Supportive** coaching expresses a belief in your capability to improve. It's positive, but not overly so.

To fully use Self-Coaching, follow these three steps:

1. **Notice** that you're at a choice point. *Nicely done*—this is the hardest part. It's okay to think these thoughts and feel these feelings right now.

2. **Choose** your goal and a tool. Decide what you really want for yourself in the long term. Pick a tool that you can use *right now* to push you in that valued direction. Write it down to make it more real.
   If you're about to avoid a task, you could:

   o Break off a chunk

   o Use a timer

   o Start a Pomodoro

   o Promise yourself a reward

   o Ask an Accountability Partner for moral support

3. **Coach** yourself. Say something to yourself that's *strategic* and *supportive*. Say it **out loud** if necessary!

Here's an example that I experience a lot. The task that I avoid the most is grading—particularly grading lengthy writing assignments. I have to pull out every tool in my Toolbox for this task, and even then I end up procrastinating on it more than I'd like.

On page 42 is what successful Self-Coaching for grading my first-year students' papers might look like.

Prepare for using Self-Coaching by filling in the chart on page 43 using your own example of a choice point that comes up a lot for you. It could be for a task you're avoiding or any other moment of emotional struggle.

You can find an additional blank version of the Self-Coaching steps worksheet at *www.guilford.com/knouse-materials*.

SELF-COACHING EXAMPLE

Self-Coaching step	
1. **Notice** that you're at a choice point and accept your thoughts and feelings.	<u>Every part of me</u> wants to stop grading papers and do something else. I'm tired. I have 10 more papers to grade, and it's taking <u>forever</u>. It's not fair that I have to do this on a sunny day when everyone else is outside having fun. The students probably won't read my feedback anyway. :(
2. **Choose** a goal and tools.	I really <u>do</u> want to make progress here. Okay, I'm going to get myself a fresh cup of coffee and put on the LoFi Beats playlist on Spotify (temptation bundling), then set a timer and commit to 4 Pomodoros of grading (Pomodoro Technique). After that, I'll go work in the yard (self-reward).
3. **Coach** yourself.	You can commit to 2 more hours, and then you'll be able to enjoy working in the yard more. Even if you don't finish all 10 papers, it'll still be a lot less to do tomorrow. You really do care about your students. You can do this.

SELF-COACHING

Self-Coaching step	
1. **Notice** that you're at a choice point and accept your thoughts and feelings.	
2. **Choose** a goal and tools.	
3. **Coach** yourself.	

3

tools for emotions and relationships

Although it's not part of the official diagnosis, most adults with ADHD experience difficulties related to their experiences with strong emotions—especially negative emotions. Although this book is not designed to help people who are experiencing full-blown emotional disorders like anxiety disorders or depression, I wanted to include strategies that can help loosen the hold emotions can have over your actions.

Many adults with ADHD also experience problems and strains in their interpersonal relationships related to their symptoms, including intimate relationships, family relationships, friendships, and parenting. So I've also included some basic strategies for getting along with other people—even though this book isn't designed to cover everything about that topic.

Moments of Mindfulness

You might associate the word *mindfulness* with meditation, silent retreats, or Buddhist monks. None of those associations is necessarily wrong, but they miss the core of what mindfulness is.

Mindfulness is paying attention to one thing, on purpose, without judgment.

In our busy, tech-filled world, there are very few moments when we're paying attention to any one thing and not evaluating whether that thing is good or bad, interesting or uninteresting, useful or useless. But research shows that finding islands of intentional focus can benefit well-being and stress reduction. There are even a few studies that used a structured mindfulness program with trained therapists to help adults with ADHD reduce their symptoms in daily life—however, we don't yet know if practicing mindfulness on your own impacts ADHD symptoms directly. What we do know is that mindfulness has plenty of other potential benefits that make it worth a try.

If you want to try out mindfulness meditation—a traditional form of mindfulness practice—plenty of free resources can help. In particular, I recommend the work of Jon Kabat-Zinn, the first person to scientifically study the benefits of mindfulness as it relates to health. Traditional mindfulness meditation exercises involve paying attention to one thing, such as your breath, and repeatedly and gently directing your attention back to it when you become distracted. The app store is a good place to start if you're interested in dipping your toe into the mindfulness meditation waters.

But if the thought of sitting quietly and focusing on your breathing sounds like torture—which it might, especially if you have ADHD—there are many other ways to incorporate mindfulness into your daily life. Here my advice is similar to my advice for exercise (page 187): The best form of mindfulness practice is the practice that you will actually do.

Let's focus on that definition of mindfulness to generate some ideas.

Mindfulness is:

- Paying attention to one thing
- On purpose
- Without judgment

Think about all the moments in your day when you are doing two or more things at once, then consider subtracting until you're down to one thing and practicing mindfulness with that activity. For example, you can:

- Go for a walk or run and spend 10 minutes of it focusing on your breathing (no music!)
- Do a household chore and spend 10 minutes of it focusing on your physical movements (no podcasts!)
- Eat your lunch while really focusing on the sensory experience of eating (no TV!)
- Have a conversation with your partner while focusing on the details of their face (no phone scrolling!)
- Sit outside for 5 minutes focusing on the sounds of the birds and wind in the trees

These bite-sized Moments of Mindfulness just might help focus your mind, help you detach from strong emotions, and pave the way for a deeper mindfulness practice. Regardless, those moments will be richer and maybe more enjoyable.

Emotional Antidotes

Strong emotions can push and pull your behavior around in ways that you might later regret. But emotions are also flexible—they respond to new experiences, moment to moment. So there are strategies you can use to change strong emotions like anger, frustration, impatience, fear, and sadness—or at least turn down the volume on these feelings so that it's easier to choose what you *actually* want to do. **Important:** The idea here isn't to push away, deny, or suppress your emotions or—even worse—to *pretend* that you feel a particular way. Rather, Emotional Antidotes are things you can do in the moment to change the intensity of your emotions, so you're freer to act in ways that are in line with your values and goals.

Ideas for Emotional Antidotes include:

- Any of the mindfulness ideas listed in the previous section.
- A video clip that cues an emotion opposite to the strong emotion—for example, a 1-minute clip of a routine from your favorite stand-up comedian or a ridiculous yet hilarious short clip from a favorite movie.*
- A song that cues a different emotion from the one you're experiencing. For example, if you're feeling anxious and full of self-doubt, maybe "Eye of the Tiger" by Survivor is your jam. Or if you're frustrated and angry, a spin of "Surfin' Bird" by the Trashmen might make you crack a smile.
- When in doubt: Dance it out.

List out any Emotional Antidotes you can think of below, and then maybe make a playlist:

_____

_____

_____

Speed Bumps

By *Speed Bumps,* I mean purposefully placing barriers between you and the ability to do things in an emotional state that you'll later regret. I'm not talking about just negative emotions here because positive emotions can also be associated with acting impulsively and doing things that aren't in your longer-term best interest.

Speed Bumps are an example of the idea of hacking the environment introduced in Chapter 2. With Speed Bumps, the idea is to hack your environment *in advance* so that you put space, time, or steps

---

*My picks: The "I'm in a glass case of emotion!" scene from *Anchorman.* Or pretty much anything from *Anchorman.*

between you and a certain action. For example, if you know you cannot be trusted around Cheetos (me!), a very effective Speed Bump would be to avoid keeping Cheetos around the house or to buy them only in tiny bags instead of party size. The table below contains some examples of actions and possible Speed Bumps for them. You can probably think of better ones!

Clear Requests

Being effective in relationships requires you to clearly communicate your wants and needs to others. Asking effectively for what you want will help others understand your reasoning and will increase the likelihood that you will get what you need or want. Communicating effectively can boost your confidence in relationships too.

Speed Bumps

Possibly regrettable action	Speed bump idea
Buying stuff online you don't need	Delete your credit card information from autofill; delete your Amazon account; keep your credit card in a safe; change your Amazon password to "doIreallyneedthis"; get rid of credit cards and use debit cards or a charge card like Fizz.
Sending angry emails to people	Create a dummy email account where you send angry emails first. If you think something is even mildly questionable (you may underestimate this when angry), send it to yourself first and wait a couple of hours before deciding to forward it on.
Drinking too much	Alternate alcoholic beverages with nonalcoholic ones and entrust a supportive friend to dole out your drinks; put a sticky note with the word *No* on your liquor, wine, or beer cabinet/fridge.

You can use this simple request formula when asking people for things in person or in writing, such as via email. This strategy is adapted from the work of Dr. Marsha Linehan and is a part of her dialectical behavior therapy program, which incorporates a broad range of cognitive-behavioral skills like the ones in this book. Just remember the acronym **DEAR:*** Describe, Express, Ask, and Reward.

- **Describe** the current situation in a clear and objective manner (no opinions; just the facts).
- **Express** your thoughts, feelings, or perspective on the situation.
- **Ask** for what you want specifically and clearly.
- **Reward** your listener. Thank them for considering your request and, if applicable, state what's in it for them.

Check out the two examples on the next page.

In my experience as the recipient of many requests from my university students, the most important part of DEAR is the *clear and specific Ask*. If there is no Ask, as the recipient of the request, I can feel like the requester is just sort of dumping a problem in my lap that I need to solve for them. A clear Ask gives a person something to respond to. Even if they don't agree, it is a starting point for negotiation.

Your turn: Decide on something you would like to ask for from a person in your life and write out your DEAR.

Describe: _____

Express: _____

Ask: _____

Reward: _____

---

*DEAR is a nice moniker for this strategy because it reminds me of the opening to a letter or email: *Dear* So-and-So.

Examples of Using DEAR

	Writing an email to your supervisor to request a schedule change: "Dear Mr. or Ms. Boss . . . "	Asking your partner for more support with child care tasks: "Hey [term of endearment] . . . "
D—Describe	Currently the days that I work until 6:00 P.M. are Monday/Wednesday. Recently my partner has needed to schedule regular health care appointments at 4:00 P.M. every other week, and I need to accompany them.	Things have gotten busier for me at work this last quarter, and I haven't had time to work out in the evenings like I used to. But I can't work out in the morning because I've got to get [kid] ready for the bus by 8:00 A.M.
E—Express	I'm concerned that these changes might interfere with my scheduled work hours, and I want to prevent that.	As you know, if I can't work out regularly, I get a little crazy!
A—Ask	I would like to request to switch the days I work until 6:00 P.M. from Monday/Wednesday to Tuesday/Thursday.	Could we choose three days during the week that you will take over getting [kid] on the bus so that I can work out?
R—Reward	I realize this change might not happen immediately due to having to adjust others' schedules, and I appreciate your considering my request. Thank you!	I want to make sure you're getting your workout time in too because I know it's important to you, so let's also discuss that. Love you!

Effective Apologies

When we have broken someone's trust or when our actions have harmed someone, apology can be an important step toward repair. Fortunately, the field of psychology is beginning to identify what makes for an Effective Apology. Psychologist Roy Lewicki and his colleagues looked at prior research and identified six possibly important components of an apology and tested them in a series of studies. These components were:

1. Express regret: Say how sorry you are for the offense
2. **Explain reasons:** Describe the reasons for the offense* *nondefensively*
3. **Acknowledge responsibility:** Demonstrate that you understand your part in the offense and its impact
4. Declare repentance: Express a commitment to not repeat the offense
5. **Offer repair:** Describe how you will fix the problem and rebuild trust
6. Request forgiveness: Ask the person you wronged to forgive you

Lewicki and colleagues discovered in their research that apologies containing more of these components were more effective than those containing fewer components. However, three components (in **boldface,** above) were especially important: explanation of **reasons** for the offense, acknowledgment of **responsibility,** and offer of **repair.** This means that, in general:

Here's how this happened, but I'm responsible and I know it hurt you. Here's what I'll do to fix it.

. . . will be more effective than:

I'm so sorry I did that. I promise never to do it again. Please forgive me.

The first apology seems more tailored to the person and situation in question, which may help it feel more sincere to the listener. And I can't help noticing that this "better" apology option shares some features with the kind of Self-Coaching recommended on page 40. Specifically, the offer of repair is focused on strategies designed to move the situation forward.

---

*We don't recommend that you use "my ADHD" as one of the reasons for your error. A more specific explanation of what went wrong can lead to better offers of repair (solutions) and possibly more understanding on the part of your listener. It also shows you have really thought about what went wrong.

Use the chart on the facing page to practice constructing an apology that contains the most important components for a current situation or one you've experienced in the past.

Of course the ultimate effective trust rebuilder is to *actually carry out the repair you have offered*. You can use the other tools in this Toolbox to help you with follow-through.

Support Communities

Support from other people is one of the most powerful psychological forces we know of. People who have gone through what you're going through can provide encouragement and empathy, but they can also share practical tips for living well with ADHD from their own experiences.

CHADD (Children and Adults with Attention-Deficit/Hyperactivity Disorder) is a U.S. national advocacy organization for people and families living with ADHD. CHADD organizes a network of affiliate Support Communities across the United States. To see if there is a community in your area, visit *https://chadd.org/affiliate-locator*. The Attention Deficit Disorder Association, which focuses on adults, offers virtual support groups and work groups for people with the disorder at *https://add.org/adda-virtual-programs*.

Your Support Communities need not be ADHD-exclusive. Think about all the groups and communities you're a part of and whether they can provide support for your efforts to cope with ADHD. If you're not sure how to ask for help, refer to the Clear Requests tool earlier in this chapter.

CONSTRUCTING AN APOLOGY

	Example: Missing a meeting	Your example:
Express regret	I'm so sorry that I missed our meeting yesterday.	
Explain what happened	My prior meeting ran overtime, and I got in my car to go home without even looking at my calendar.	
Acknowledge responsibility and harm	This was clearly my fault, and I know it wasn't respectful of the time you had set aside for us to meet.	
Offer repair	If you're willing, I'd like to reschedule at a time that's convenient for you, and this time I will set three reminders in my Google calendar!	

PART TWO

menu of moves for living well

This part of the book is a true *choose your own adventure* of living better with ADHD. Each chapter addresses a specific challenge you might be struggling with and directs you to possible skills and solutions, including tools from the Toolbox. Most chapters in the Menu begin with questions you'll answer to zero in on your specific needs and get information tailored to your situation. How do you decide which chapter to start with? You might choose an area that causes the most problems for you. Alternatively, you could choose an area that's less challenging for you but one that you think will be easier to tackle. (An early "win" can be a good thing.) No matter what, take things one step at a time and pace yourself. You'll probably have to try out different solutions and tweak them to fit your life. This is all part of the process.

4

show up on time

"As a person with ADHD, I have an insanely different relationship
with time than others."

Dr. Barkley coined the term *time blindness* for the struggles people with
ADHD experience perceiving and managing time. Those struggles
may have shown up for you in terms of getting yourself where you
need to be when you need to be there. For many adults with ADHD,
showing up late can be a chronic problem that becomes a source of
stress and conflict in relationships. Although people and cultures have
different ideas about what counts as "on time" and it's not helpful to get
too judgmental about this issue, if you've decided to read this chapter,
it probably means that being late is something that's causing problems
for you and that it's something you'd like to improve.

Maybe you feel like you're stressed out by consistently running
behind with no time to prepare, to *breathe*. Or maybe you feel like
you're letting others down or being judged negatively for showing
up late. And perhaps you've even missed out on some opportunities
because of chronic lateness. Whatever the case, it can be really stressful to feel like you're always "the late person," and it can also feel like
something that you can't possibly change. But showing up somewhere
at a specific time is, like any behavior, something you can change with
the right strategies and by practicing those strategies until they become
a habit—even if you have ADHD. To identify which strategies might

be the most helpful for you, begin by completing the self-assessment below.

At the same time, changing long-standing behaviors can be hard, and sometimes you need support. As always, if the ideas in this chapter seem like they could be helpful but you just can't seem to implement them consistently on your own, you might benefit from working with a cognitive-behavioral therapist who can support your efforts.

Self-Assessment and Roadmap

Read each statement below and on the next page and choose the best answer for you by putting a checkmark (✓) in the box. Use your answers to choose which sections to review.

- *A lot* like me!—Definitely review this section!
- Somewhat like me—Review this section if you need additional ideas.
- Not like me—This section doesn't seem to apply to you, so skip it if you want.

	Not like me	Somewhat like me	*A lot* like me!	Sections to review
I realize only at the last minute (if at all) that I'm supposed to be somewhere else.				A (page 59)
I get really absorbed in doing something and then end up leaving late for appointments.				B (page 59)
I don't allow enough time to get ready to leave and/ or to get where I'm going.				C (page 60)

	Not like me	Somewhat like me	*A lot* like me!	Sections to review
The thought of showing up too early for something makes me feel uncomfortable or like I'd be wasting time.				D (page 61)
I'm a human being, which means no matter what, I'm going to be late from time to time.				E (page 62)

≫ A: I realize only at the last minute (if at all) that I'm supposed to be somewhere else.

Without knowing where you're supposed to be, it'll be impossible to be on time throughout your day. If this describes you:

❑ Develop and consistently use a Calendar System (page 16).

You can use this to keep track of appointments and keep yourself on track in the process. If you choose an electronic calendar, you can add reminders and locations to each appointment. Honestly, now that I'm in my 40s, I have *no idea* what I'm supposed to be doing an hour from now without looking at my Google calendar.

≫ B: I get really absorbed in doing something and then end up leaving late.

Like many adults with ADHD, you may experience that state of "hyperfocus" where you're so absorbed in a task that you don't realize time is flying by. Or perhaps you're working on something and do realize you need to leave soon but think to yourself, "I can just finish *this one thing* before I leave . . . ," and then you've given yourself 5 minutes to make a 15-minute trip. If so, you can try these ideas:

❏ Wear a watch and put more clocks around your house in strategic locations (page 22).

❏ Set a timer with an alarm before starting on a hyperfocus-prone task (page 23).

❏ Add reminders to the appointments on your calendar that "ping" 60 minutes before the appointment, 30 before, and so on (page 23).

❏ Use a Choice Point Analysis (page 36) to notice the thoughts you're having that are giving you permission to keep doing what you're doing (and delay leaving), then use Self-Coaching (page 40).

❏ See Chapter 11 for additional ideas for managing hyperfocus states.

>> C: I don't allow enough time to get ready to leave and/or to get where I'm going.

ADHD can affect your perception of time—how quickly it passes and how much you'll need to accomplish tasks. You might be late sometimes because you don't allow enough preparation, transition, or travel time before an appointment or event. To address this problem, you could certainly:

❏ Add reminders to the appointments on your calendar that "ping" 60 minutes before the appointment, 30 before, and so on (page 23).

But I'm also going to suggest that you go one better and actually:

❏ Block out what you *think* will be an overestimate of required transition time by adding "Transition Time" as an event in your calendar.

In other words, you're going to make that transition time a place-holding reality in your Calendar System so that you give it the time it deserves. And you're going to purposefully overestimate that time so you can correct for any difficulties with time perception. (Don't worry—over time, if you engage in this practice, you'll probably get a more accurate sense of how much time is actually needed.)

I started using this strategy after years of forcing myself to rush to (and be sweaty at) my first appointment of the day on mornings when I teach fitness classes (Jazzercise, to be specific). Despite teaching the same schedule week after week, I had the time block for my class *ending at the time the class ended,* and then I had to rely on my own (limited) memory and awareness to allow time to drive home, shower (when I remembered to leave enough time for it), and travel to work before the next scheduled event. Nowadays the event "Teach Jazzercise" is *always* followed in my calendar by an event 1 hour and 15 minutes long labeled "Travel/Shower/Travel." A simple fix that has greatly improved my quality of life—not to mention my personal hygiene.

Take a look at your calendar. Can you identify spots where a "Transition Time" event is needed to set yourself up for success? If so, add an event and make sure to overestimate how much time you'll need.

≫ D: The thought of showing up too early for something makes me feel uncomfortable or like I'd be wasting time.

For some people with ADHD, the idea of having to wait for something can feel excruciating and bring up anxiety or just generally icky feelings. If this is true for you, it might be contributing to your problems with lateness because your efforts to avoid having to wait and "waste time" actually end up making you late. If you suspect this might apply to you, you can try to:

❑ Identify things you can do with extra time while waiting (so you won't feel like you're "wasting" it).

In her work, psychologist and ADHD expert Dr. Mary Solanto refers to such chunks of open, unoccupied time as "time cracks" and suggests that clients can think ahead and make a list of things that can be done in these small, sometimes unexpected little time-gifts. Also, the ubiquity of smartphones can certainly make it easier to access time crack activity options. Adapting this idea, you could use a time crack to:

- Check and answer emails
- Read a book or listen to a podcast or audiobook
- Do a mindfulness or relaxation exercise
- Curate your task list or preview what's next on your calendar
- Call or text with a family member or friend you've been wanting to connect with

Try making a list of your own possible time crack activities below:

_____

_____

_____

Once you've got some ideas for how you could spend any wait time that occurs, you can:

☐ Use a Choice Point Analysis (page 36) to notice thoughts and feelings that come up when you think about being early and having to wait and then use Self-Coaching (page 40).

For example, if you experience the thought "Ugh, I don't want to get there *early*—what a waste of time!" you could respond with a thought like "You know what? I'm going to leave now, so I don't have to rush and get all stressed out. And if I do get there early, I can [fill in time crack activity here] while I'm waiting."

>> E: I'm a human being, which means no matter what, I'm going to be late from time to time.

Sometimes you'll be late. It's a fact of life. Regardless of whether you have ADHD, and even if you've planned ahead and used all of these strategies meticulously (or at least given them a try), there are going to be times when you're running behind. (Just ask my hairstylist. Or my students.) What can you do? I recommend the following:

- Stop to take a deep breath. This is not the end of the world. You are not a bad person.

- Communicate with any relevant people that you will be late and when you think you'll arrive.

  As soon as you know you will likely be late, text or call the person you will be meeting or the office and let them know when you think you will arrive. (**Note:** Do not do this while driving!) Be prepared to hear that you might need to reschedule. That's okay! It's better to know this now and for the person who's expecting you to know the situation.

- Express gratitude when you arrive.

  Acknowledge the person who has waited or made accommodations for you by saying something like "Thank you so much for waiting" or "Thank you for your flexibility and grace!" It's also okay to apologize for being late; however, expressing gratitude as well can engender positive feelings.

5

remember and remember to do things

"My thoughts are like billiard balls. If a new one comes in, it knocks the previous one out of the way. Writing things on the back of my hand will bring it back to mind at least for a couple of hours. Also, I find a pocket-sized diary is helpful to remind myself of what tasks I need to prioritize for that week, so I keep a pen in my right pants pocket and a pocket diary in my left. These are my constant companions."

Forgetting can show up for people with ADHD in a few different ways. You may forget to do things when you need to do them—something psychologists call a *prospective memory failure*. You might forget that certain events are happening and so miss the opportunity to prepare for them. Or you might have trouble holding in mind information that you need to complete a task. (What did I walk into this room for?) If keeping information in mind to guide your behavior is a struggle for you, this chapter covers some strategies that might help.

Self-Assessment and Roadmap

Read each statement below and choose the best answer for you by putting a checkmark (✓) in the box. Use your answers to choose which sections to review.

- *A lot* like me!—Definitely review this section!

- Somewhat like me—Review this section if you need additional ideas.

- Not like me—This section doesn't seem to apply to you, so skip it if you want.

	Not like me	Somewhat like me	*A lot* like me!	Sections to review
I forget to do daily tasks like take my medicine or pack my lunch.				A (page 66)
It seems like I'm constantly surprised by events I forgot were happening (for example, appointments).				B (page 67)
I have trouble remembering key pieces of information, like dates, ID numbers, and passwords.				C (page 68)
I forget what I want to say in important conversations.				D (page 68)
I'm a human being, which means no matter what, I'm going to forget things.				E (page 69)

» A: I forget to do daily tasks like take my medicine or pack my lunch.

❑ Schedule the task daily in your calendar and set an alarm for it.

This is a version of the idea of Strategic Task Scheduling (page 31). The scheduling will help to ensure you've slotted the task into your day, and then the alarm will cue you to do it.

❑ Use reminders in your environment (page 23).

Use a sticky note or notecard to make a colorful, attractive reminder sign for the task you need to accomplish and put it somewhere that you'll see it at the time you need to do the task. For example: "Take your meds and have a great day!" on your bathroom mirror or "Did you pack your lunch yet?" on your bedside lamp (if you want to pack lunch the night before).

❑ Set up prompts in your environment (page 23).

In the Toolbox, we defined prompts as objects in the physical environment that cue your behavior. The idea is to lay out your environment in a way that nudges the action you want. For example, you could try putting your medication bottle right next to the handle of the faucet or—better yet—next to the toilet paper roll so that you'll see it when you engage with those parts of the environment. (Of course, wash your hands before taking your meds. ☺) You could use an "S" hook to hang your lunch bag to the handle of the refrigerator so that it's right there when it's time to pack your lunch. Get creative!

❑ Pair the frequently forgotten behavior with a more consistent one.

The technical term for this strategy is *yoking*. First think of something you almost *always* do at the time and in the place where you want the oft-forgotten behavior to occur. Next think of a way that you can use that consistent behavior to prompt the inconsistent one.

For example, if you're great at consistently brushing your teeth each morning but forgetful about your meds, you can try duct-taping your med bottle to the handle of your toothbrush or to your toothpaste tube. If you're great about remembering to feed your dog in the evening—because he **will** remind you—you can put a reminder note on the dog food bag to cue your lunch making. Maybe something like "You've fed Fido. But have you fed the You of Tomorrow?"

» B: It seems like I'm constantly surprised by events I forgot were happening (for example, appointments).

❑ Commit or recommit to the Calendar System (page 16).

I sound like a broken record, but these tools are absolutely foundational to being able to manage your ADHD. Without them, it will be hard to layer on other strategies. People sometimes get tripped up because they start to think things like "Well, I don't need to put *every-thing* in my calendar; I'll probably remember this one," which can lead to backsliding on entering appointments, missing things, and then giving up on the calendar altogether. If thoughts like this are getting in the way of committing to the calendar habit, check out the Choice Point Analysis (page 36) and effective Self-Coaching (page 40) in Chapter 2.

❑ Add in-advance alarms to unusual or especially important calendar events.

Set up pings 24 hours in advance *and* a few hours in advance for any appointments or other crucial calendar events.

❑ Post a Household Events Calendar to keep everyone on the same page.

Hang up a weekly or monthly wipe-off calendar where you can visually display upcoming events. I recommend one that's also magnetic, so you can stick needed documents to it and use magnetic hooks or clips to suspend needed objects from. At the start of each week or month, sit down with those in your household (or just yourself!) and write out all the important events for that time period.

›› C: I have trouble remembering key pieces of information, like dates, ID numbers, and passwords.

❑ Designate a specific spot in your planner or on your task list where you write down key pieces of oft-forgotten information.

This is a *no sticky note* situation! You want to be able to find the information later, so be strategic about where you'll write it. For example, I have a stack of cards on my Trello board (see page 19) labeled "Useful Links and Notes" that contains information like passwords, any instructions I've had to look up repeatedly, or other information that I just can't seem to hold in my brain.

❑ Use your phone to take pictures of information you need to remember.

Make sure your photos back up to the cloud, then create a photo album where you'll keep all these info-pictures—things like your license plate, a photo of a list of family birthdays or anniversaries, or a password list. I have an album on my Google Photos called "Laura's Memory" where I keep photos of information like this. The photo strategy could also work for learning people's names. Last semester I took a photo of each student holding up a card with their name on the first day of class and then used the photos to quiz myself to learn their names more quickly. Might be worth a shot if you are a person who struggles to learn names!

›› D: I forget what I want to say in important conversations.

It can be a painful experience to really want to express yourself and then lose your train of thought. This happens to most people from time to time, but it might be more difficult for you as a person with ADHD. Here are some strategies for saying what you need to say.

❑ Write or speak it out beforehand.

If you know that you will need to speak in class, at a meeting, or in an important conversation with a friend or loved one, it's a good idea to sort out your thoughts in advance. You can jot down a few notes or use a voice memo app on your phone to get your thoughts out into the world ahead of time.

❑ Use your notes.

It's totally okay to use notes to help prompt you during a conversation. Just explain that you really want to make sure you can express yourself, so you wrote down a few things you want to be sure to say.

❑ Rehearse it.

It might seem goofy to sit alone and talk to yourself, but if you can practice what you want to say a few times, you'll be more likely to remember it when you need to.

❑ Take a moment.

If you lose your train of thought, that's okay! Most people listening to you want you to do well and want to understand you, so don't assume anyone is judging you for needing a moment. Just say, "I'm sorry, there's something I wanted to say, and I can't quite pull it up. I'm going to take a moment and see if it comes to me." If after taking a moment you can't recall what you wanted to say, simply thank them for waiting and move on to the next point, letting them know that you'll check back with them when you remember your forgotten point.

» E: I'm a human being, which means no matter what, I'm going to forget things.

It's true, and yet it can be hard not to be pessimistic or hard on yourself when you forget something really important. When you discover you've forgotten something that has an impact on others, don't avoid communicating with them about it. Apologize sincerely (Effective Apologies, page 50) and try to make things right. Embrace the idea that you did the best that you could with what you had at the time, then engage with Self-Coaching (page 40) to identify solutions for the future and to encourage yourself toward them.

6

keep track of your stuff

"I used to be terrible at losing stuff. Now when I leave home, I check my pocket for my phone, before I step out and again after I step out the door. This has become second nature after so much practice, and I very rarely forget it anymore."

Keeping track of stuff and having the right stuff when you need it is often a struggle for adults with ADHD. "Stuff" includes digital documents and pieces of information that you need to track and organize as well. If you struggle with finding things when you need them or having what you need when you need it, you've come to the right place.

Self-Assessment and Roadmap

Read each statement on the next page and choose the best answer for you by putting a checkmark ✓) in the box. Use your answers to choose which sections to review.

- *A lot* like me!—Definitely review this section!

- Somewhat like me—Review this section if you need additional ideas.

- Not like me—This section doesn't seem to apply to you, so skip it if you want.

	Not like me	Somewhat like me	*A lot* like me!	Sections to review
I leave items somewhere in the house and then can't find them.				A (page 72)
I leave items somewhere out in the world and can't find them.				B (page 75)
I leave the house without necessary items.				C (page 76)
I lose important papers or pieces of mail.				D (page 77)
I have trouble finding important files on my computer.				E (page 78)
I'm a human, which means no matter what, I'm going to lose things sometimes.				F (page 79)

≫ A: I leave items somewhere in the house and then can't find them.

If you spend way too much time wandering around the house looking for your phone (guilty!), wallet, laptop, gym bag, or other crucial items, here are some strategies to try.

❑ Use Home Bases.

Put a basket, bin, or set of hooks just inside your front door and dump your keys, wallet, or phone there as soon as you come through the door. Put a dish or shot glass next to the sink and put your rings there when you take them off to wash the dishes. Create similar spots in your work office, if you have one, or designate a spot in your bag or backpack where your keys, phone, or other object will "live." Of course, you'll need to get in the habit of consistently putting that object in that specific spot, but over time this will become an automatic behavior, and you'll know where to look—or at least look first—when trying to locate important objects.

❑ Learn to use "find my device" features.

Apple's Find My network and Google's Find My Device networks can be a godsend if you're a chronic phone loser. (Not that you're a loser . . . you know what I mean!) You can use any device attached to your account to locate other devices on that account.

❑ Attach electronic tags to important nonelectronic objects.

AirTag (for Apple users), MotoTag (for Android), and lots of other brands of Bluetooth-enabled tags offer a handy system to locate lost nonelectronic objects like your gym bag, backpack, purse, keys, or wallet—including when you misplace things inside your house. My husband—in a not-so-subtle bid to get me to stop running frantically around the house looking for my Jazzercise bag—gifted me a set of Tile trackers and, as a Google person, I'm excited to try MotoTags, which integrate with Google's Find My Device network.

❑ Keep a list of the places you find your missing items.

Get a sticky note and write down the places you've found your missing items in the past and put that on your bathroom mirror or someplace similar. Remember that time your phone fell between the mattress and the bed frame? It might happen again. Did you leave the phone on a little shelf in the bathroom because you were listening to podcasts in the shower and then left it there? That's probably going to happen again. If you can give the You of the Future clues on where to look next time, you might reduce the time and frustration of the search.*

❑ Use what makes the missing object stand out from the environment to guide your search.

My colleague at the University of Richmond, Dr. Arryn Robbins, is an expert in the psychology of searching the visual environment and has shared some great ideas here (thanks, Dr. Robbins!). Based on her advice, before you start searching for an object, think about what makes it stand out from its environment in terms of size, color, texture, or other features. For example, if you're looking for a piece of jewelry on a carpeted floor, the shininess of the jewelry is something you can focus on as you scan the floor to make the object pop out of its environment.

❑ Act out the movements that probably took place when you lost the item.

What I mean here is to retrace your steps *and* retrace the actions that you might have taken when the item was lost. For example, if you can't find your phone but you know you had it when you pulled into your driveway, go back to the car, sit in it, and act out all the motions you would have gone through from that point forward. Putting yourself physically back in the environment and retracing your actions might help you identify possible spots where the item could be.

❑ Do a grid search.

If you are really in a missing item pickle, Dr. Robbins recommends mentally dividing the search space into a grid and systematically searching from the top row, sweeping downward. That way you will be sure you've looked everywhere, even in a messy environment. Be

---

*Also, check your car.

sure to take a deep breath first so that anxiety doesn't cause you to skip over anything!

≫ B: I leave items somewhere out in the world and can't find them.

Ugh! That time when your around-the-house search for an object leaves you with the sinking feeling that your item may be somewhere out in the world. Here are some strategies to prevent this from happening or help you locate items when it does.

❑ Use "find my device" features and electronic tags.

See the description in Section A (page 73). These electronic aids can help you locate important objects where you left them.

❑ Develop a checking routine for important items.

This idea came from one of my former clients. He cultivated the habit of running his hands over his front pants pockets every time he stood up so that he could verify that his phone or wallet was "on him." The same could be done if you designate a Home Base (page 72) for key items in your purse or backpack. If you practice this physical motion that allows you to check for an item, it will eventually become unconscious and automatic.

❑ Buy only inexpensive versions of items you might lose.

Try to follow this rule: *Don't take items out of the house that you can't afford to lose.* Think $5 sunglasses and $10 umbrellas. And—for crying out loud!—skip the AirPods and buy vastly cheaper versions that won't set you back hundreds of dollars if you lose them. (I don't have ADHD, and I'm 100% certain that *I cannot be trusted* with AirPods.) Consider getting cubic zirconia versions of your precious gemstone jewelry for everyday wear. You can keep the genuine articles in a safe place, and you'll have gained some additional peace of mind.

» C: I leave the house without necessary items.

Here are some strategies if you keep forgetting to take what you need along with you.

- ❑ Use a Home Base (page 72) in your home or at your office.
- ❑ Add the needed item to the title of the appointment in your calendar.

For example: "***Bring gift:*** Lunch with Angie" can help you remember to grab that random gift you bought for Angie before you leave the house instead of just relying on yourself to remember. Better yet, add an alarm to this calendar event for 10 minutes before you're supposed to leave the house, and it becomes a reminder message that will literally pop up in front of your face.

- ❑ Use a Go Bag (or Box).

This is a riff on the idea of the Home Base. Get a cheap reusable grocery bag and hang it on the doorknob of the door you always leave the house from, *or*, if it's a box, place it directly in front of the door so that you have to move the box to open the door. Put anything in the Go Bag/Box that you need to take with you the next time you leave the house. **Important:** *Don't actually take the bag/box with you, just its contents* so that the Go Bag/Box stays by the door to use next time.

- ❑ Use a Go List.

Stick a cheap whiteboard at eye level on the inside of the door you leave by. Write any items or reminders you need before leaving the house there, right in your face.

>> D: I lose important papers or pieces of mail.

Where *did* you put that permission slip for your kid's field trip? Or that Bath & Body Works coupon you really wanted to use? While many documents have moved to digital in the past several years, we're still far away from that paperless society I've been hearing about since the 1980s. Here are some tips to prevent the losing of papers.

❑ Take pictures of all important documents with your phone immediately after acquiring them.

Then add the photos to a digital folder or album titled something like "Important Papers," so you have those images all in one place. Even if you can't fill out the forms electronically, you may be able to print them out or write and sign a note—in the case of a permission slip—covering all the information. If they're clear enough, photos of barcodes from coupons will scan just like the real thing.

❑ Have one and only one "dump spot" for all mail and papers you need to review.

Get a basket or document tray for mail and any documents you haven't yet taken a picture of or reviewed. On a regular basis—schedule it in your Calendar System (page 16) or use Rewarding Consequences to motivate yourself (page 29)—go through the things in the tray and either throw them out, take a picture of them, or do what you need to do to respond to or process the item.

❑ Stick important papers to your Household Events Calendar (page 152).

In Chapter 5 (page 67) we suggested using a large magnetic wipe-off calendar to display important events for the week or month as a reminder to everyone in the household about what's coming up. If you have one of these, you can stick important documents related to calendar events—for example, a permission slip—to the calendar, so you'll have them when you need them.

≫ E: I have trouble finding important files on my computer.

If you find yourself constantly on the hunt for an important PDF, email, or .doc file you really need, here are some ideas for preventing document misplacement or finding documents efficiently.

❑ Don't dump—create a *simple* file structure.

Try to avoid just dumping everything on your desktop or downloading to your Downloads folder and leaving everything in there. Create a simple file structure for the categories of documents you use most frequently. You can add subfolders, but don't make an overly complicated structure that is too clunky and complicated to use. Instead, let your needs guide the structure—that is, when you find you *need* a new folder or subfolder for an actual document, create it then rather than trying to make a structure you *think* will be useful.

❑ Name files so that they're easily searchable.

The experts refer to this as having *naming conventions,* and the point is to create file names that will help you identify and locate files later. Instead of "receipt17.000236624," name your files using more specifics such as, "Knouse gas receipt 7.22.24." In particular, the date can be very helpful in retracing your digital steps.

❑ Learn the search features for your email, computer, or cloud storage platform.

These days your computer, email program, and file storing and sharing platforms like Google Docs or Dropbox probably all have robust search features. Take time to teach yourself how to use them and you'll prevent future frustration. Thinking of likely words in the file title and limiting the search by dates or file type can help you locate things faster.

» F: I'm a human, which means no matter what, I'm going to lose things sometimes.

If you have ADHD, there are just going to be times when you lose things. And that can be pretty frustrating. As mentioned earlier, consider reducing the potential impact of misplacing things by buying inexpensive versions of items you might lose. In other words, don't take items out of your house that you can't afford to lose. Some more ideas for reducing the impact of losing electronic devices follow.

❑ Set up syncing of your phone contacts, calendar, and task list information.

That way, if you misplace your phone, you won't lose access to this key information.

❑ Set up syncing of files on your device to a cloud storage platform.

This is a best practice for preventing data loss in general, and it can also save you headaches if you lose your phone or laptop. And finally:

❑ It's ultimately just stuff. Take it easy on yourself.

Being an adult in the "modern world" involves managing so many physical objects and pieces of information that it's no surprise that folks with (and without) ADHD struggle to manage it all. If you lose something important, try your best to approach yourself with compassion and good Self-Coaching (page 40).

7

plan and prioritize

"I prefer to just wing it. I am deciding on the spot what I need to do next and not worrying about what I need to do three or five steps out. This works for some things I need to do, but for others it's a disaster because events and deadlines are arriving sooner than I expected, and I haven't even gotten to step 1, 2, or 3 in trying to prepare for them. The future slams into me like a rogue wave I didn't see coming."

Getting to a meaningful goal takes multiple small actions spread out and coordinated across time. If you have problems planning out the necessary steps toward a big, complicated goal or problems coordinating your efforts across multiple goals, this is the section for you.

Self-Assessment and Roadmap

Read each statement on page the facing page and choose the best answer for you by putting a checkmark (✓) in the box. Use your answers to choose which sections to review.

- *A lot* like me!—Definitely review this section!
- Somewhat like me—Review this section if you need additional ideas.
- Not like me—This section doesn't seem to apply to you, so skip it if you want.

	Not like me	Somewhat like me	*A lot* like me!	Sections to review
I have trouble recognizing when it's necessary to plan out something.				A (page 81)
I have trouble making step-by-step plans toward a big goal.				B (page 82)
I have trouble deciding what's most important and how to spend my time.				C (page 84)
I'm a human, which means no matter what, I'll sometimes fail to plan ahead or spend my time on less important things.				D (page 84)

≫ A: I have trouble recognizing when it's necessary to plan out something.

❏ Set up a Calendar System (page 16).

First, you'll need to have a Calendar System in operation so that you can realize when "big things" are coming up.

❏ Use a Task-Tracking System (page 17).

Next, you'll need to bring a Task-Tracking System online so that you can coordinate your efforts across all the necessary steps.

❏ Ask yourself: Could I get this done in an hour?

If the answer is a big *no*, then it probably means the task will require breaking down and planning out. Here are some examples of tasks that will require planning:

- Social events such as parties or other get-togethers
- Home improvement and gardening projects
- Trips and vacations
- Choosing and enrolling in an educational program
- Finding a job
- Doing your taxes
- Signing your child up for day care, school, or extracurricular programs
- Work or school projects and papers

If you see any of these things on the horizon, you'll want to star, circle, highlight, and underline that task in your list! Then read the next section.

›› B: I have trouble making step-by-step plans toward a big goal.

Okay, you know you *need* a plan, but you can't quite get there. Try these suggestions to get unstuck.

❑ Use Task Chunks (page 28).

No matter what, planning is going to require breaking a big task into smaller steps. If you haven't read the section on Task Chunks in Chapter 2, do that first and come back here.

❑ Read the instructions.

If your plan involves interacting with institutions—like workplaces, schools, government agencies—first read up on any requirements these agencies have and what the processes are for you to get what you want from them. Then you can make sure your plan includes these steps.

❑ Make it physical and visual.

You're probably not going to be able to hold all the information contained in your grand plan in your head. Create a space to organize your ideas in a way that you can put them outside your brain and move them in space. For example, get a big magnetic whiteboard to map out your ideas and move things around or use sticky notes on a wall so that you can adjust as you think through your plan. Virtual bulletin boards like Miro or Google's Jamboard are also great tools for mapping out ideas with many moving parts. Just make sure that once you've got the steps of your plan, you put these steps into your Task-Tracking System.

❑ Storyboard and simulate.

If you think about it, a good plan is sort of like a story that unfolds toward its conclusion. If you find it hard to plan things in the abstract, trying making things more real by telling yourself the story of how you will get from point A to point B. You could even draw pictures, make diagrams, or close your eyes and imagine events unfolding if that's helpful to you.

And just like a good story, executing your plan is going to involve barriers and challenges for you, the hero. Ask yourself what obstacles could arise and how you can plan to manage them. For example, imagine a parent wants to achieve the daunting goal of enrolling a child in day care. The parent could tell the following story to themselves or talk it out with their partner:

First, I think about what kinds of things I'm looking for in a day care and write down a list. Then I get curious about what the options are in my area. Next, I go online and search for locations that are close to my house or my work. Hmm, that's going to get complicated fast. Okay, so I'll make an online doc where I can record the information about the different day cares and maybe rate them based on what I'm looking for? Then after that I should talk to my partner, and we can figure out which one to apply to. Hmm . . . although my friend told me it's hard to get a slot sometimes, so I should probably pick more than one option. Maybe top 3? Okay, then I see I'll need to look up how to apply to them . . .

❑ Talk it out.

It can be easier to plan if you're getting out of your head and discussing it with another person. This might be a great time for an Accountability Partner (page 33), a counselor, or a coach (see the Resources). Or you can ask a friend or family member to be your sounding board as you plan the important steps toward your goal. Then offer to do the same for them.

» C: I have trouble deciding what's most important and how to spend my time.

With multiple competing priorities, it can be hard to decide what to tackle first. It's often the most important tasks that trigger the unpleasant emotions, causing us to veer toward easier, safer, less important tasks. Read or revisit these Toolbox items for help in prioritizing:

❑ Priority Labeling (or Sorting) (page 18)
❑ Choice Point Analysis (page 36) and Self-Coaching (page 40)

» D: I'm a human, which means no matter what, I'll sometimes fail to plan ahead or spend my time on less important things.

You may have found yourself in a spot where, looking back, you should have planned ahead better or spent your time in a different way. Maybe someone is frustrated with you or you're really frustrated with yourself. Maybe it feels like this has happened so often that things can never change. These thoughts and feelings are understandable, but they're just thoughts and feelings. They don't determine your future, and they don't determine who you are. When you're ready, take some time to look back using a Choice Point Analysis (page 36) and see if you can identify any skills or strategies you could use the next time to make things better. Then engage with Self-Coaching (page 40) to lock it in.

8

complete tasks accurately

"I waste time daydreaming, mind wandering, or just getting distracted by some 'shiny thing.' Then I realize that the project is due very soon and I haven't set aside enough time to do it right. So I now have to rush through it to meet the deadline and much of what I have done doesn't really fulfill the task I was given."

Let's face it—being an adult involves navigating some very tedious and bureaucratic processes that can be extra-challenging when you have ADHD. If you have difficulty following complex instructions accurately or problems missing details in your work or other pursuits, this chapter is for you.

Self-Assessment and Roadmap

Read each statement on the next page and choose the best answer for you by putting a checkmark (✓) in the box. Use your answers to choose which sections to review.

- *A lot* like me!—Definitely review this section!
- Somewhat like me—Review this section if you need additional ideas.
- Not like me—This section doesn't seem to apply to you, so skip it if you want.

	Not like me	Somewhat like me	*A lot* like me!	Sections to review
I skip important parts of my work or don't follow all the directions.				A (page 86)
I lose focus in the middle of the task and miss things I should do.				B (page 87)
I rush through tedious tasks to get them over with as soon as possible.				C (page 87)
I'm a human being, which means no matter what, I'm going to make mistakes in my work at times.				D (page 88)

» A: I skip important parts of my work or don't follow all the directions.

I see this all the time as a college professor: A smart student with good ideas misses big chunks of what's required on an assignment. This might not end up being a big deal on a college assignment, but in other situations it could have serious consequences. Maybe you've experienced the consequences of this problem in your life. If so, here are some strategies to try:

- ❑ Engineer and use your Reduced-Distraction Environment (page 25).
- ❑ Before you start, write out the directions in your own words, step by step, checklist style.

Sometimes directions are very poorly written or confusing and hard to follow. When you write them in your own words, they are clearer to you and broken down into those manageable chunks I keep emphasizing (page 28). If the directions are in electronic format, you could copy/paste each step into a numbered list to help you focus on each one. Then check them off as you complete them.

❑ When you *think* you've finished, read the directions again and adjust as necessary.

Because I was born in the 1980s, I often describe this strategy using the words of a popular rap icon from that era who warned that checking oneself is a good way to avoid wrecking oneself.

❑ Get an Accountability Partner (page 33) who's willing to give your work the once-over.

Simply knowing that someone else will look at your work might also motivate you to check over more than you would otherwise.

≫ B: I lose focus in the middle of the task and miss things I should do.

❑ Engineer and use your Reduced-Distraction Environment (page 25).
❑ Use the Pomodoro Technique to stay focused and motivated (page 32).
❑ Use Strategic Task Scheduling (page 31) to optimize the time that you work on the task and build in Rewarding Consequences (page 29).

≫ C: I rush through tedious tasks to get them over with as soon as possible.

Maybe doing detail-oriented work *feels* icky, so you sacrifice accuracy for getting it over with. If so, here are some ideas to try.

❑ Try temptation bundling (Rewarding Consequences, page 29).

If it's not too distracting, choose your very favorite musical artist, playlist, Broadway show, or genre and allow yourself to listen to that music *only* when you're doing a task that feels super icky.

❑ Estimate the time you think you will need to complete the task, *double that,* and set a timer (page 22). Add a Rewarding Consequence (page 29) at the end.

This strategy will force you to spend more time on the task than you think you'll need. If you get done before the timer goes off, use that time to reread the directions and go back over your work.

» D: I'm a human being, which means no matter what, I'm going to make mistakes in my work at times.

You might be in a spot right now where rushing through something or missing important steps has caused you problems or upset people who are important to you. It might feel like you should just give up because there's no way you're ever going to be able to do better. These thoughts and feelings are *real,* but they're not *true.* They don't determine your future. When your mistakes impact other people, make a sincere apology (Effective Apologies, page 50) and revisit the strategies in this section to see how you could do better next time. And, as always, develop the kind of Self-Coaching (page 40) that can encourage you forward.

9

get started
and restarted

"A few years back, a good friend of mine said he was getting a bit tired of constantly giving me roadmaps to help with my problems that I never wanted to follow. I remember thinking, 'I have a million of those maps in my head. I know how to make them. What I need to know is how, as the navigator, I get the driver to follow my instructions instead of f★★★ing off to the river to throw rocks at fish.'"

Procrastination is among the most common problems faced by adults with ADHD—one that can block you from reaching your meaningful goals and cause stress in your life. Being an adult involves daily competition between short-term payoffs and longer-term accomplishments (and requirements). It might feel like procrastination is just a part of you—like something that's so ingrained that you can't change it. But psychologists actually know a lot about why we procrastinate and what strategies help people get unstuck.

One reason procrastination can be such a tough nut to crack is that people procrastinate at different times for different reasons. So part of getting unstuck is gaining a better understanding of what's causing *your* avoidance in specific situations.

Self-Assessment and Roadmap

Read each statement below and choose the best answer for you by putting a checkmark (✓) in the box. Use your answers to choose which sections to review.

- *A lot* like me!—Definitely review this section!
- Somewhat like me—Review this section if you need additional ideas.
- Not like me—This section doesn't seem to apply to you, so skip it if you want.

	Not like me	Somewhat like me	*A lot* like me!	Sections to review
I don't have a good idea of what really needs to be done, so I spend time on less important tasks.				A (page 91)
I look at big tasks on my task list or think about them and instantly feel overwhelmed and then avoid.				B (page 91)
I find myself doing everything *except* the thing I should be doing.				C (page 92)
When I think about doing something I'm avoiding, I have a lot of negative thoughts, *or* I think things like "I'll have more time to do it later."				D (page 94)
I'm a human being, which means no matter what, sometimes I'm going to procrastinate.				E (page 94)

≫ A: I don't have a good idea of what really needs to be done, so I spend time on less important tasks.

First, you need to set up a:

❑ Task-Tracking System (page 17)

If you haven't committed to this foundational tool for fighting procrastination, now is the time. Be sure to also use:

❑ Priority Labeling (or Sorting) (page 18)

Practice applying the A/B/C priority labels to the items on your list. Remember, those A tasks are ones you need to work on immediately, but the runner-up B tasks probably involve small pieces that could also be A tasks. And if those A tasks still just seem too overwhelming, read on.

≫ B: I look at big tasks on my task list or think about them and instantly feel overwhelmed and then avoid.

This makes emotional sense—we tend to avoid those things that trigger negative emotions, and this avoidance can happen without much thinking or even awareness. When this happens, use:

❑ Task Chunks (page 28)

Chunking up tasks will allow you to create less overwhelming micro-tasks. These smaller Task Chunks can help you get unstuck by reducing your sense of task dread and giving you a little hit of achievement for checking them off your list. Your big, scary A task becomes a series of smaller, less scary and more specific A chunks. Here's something to keep in mind: It's okay to create a chunk that seems absurdly small.

For example, despite being an extrovert, I despise making phone calls unless it's for a fun, social purpose.* To get myself moving, I will often tell myself, "Okay, you JUST have to look up so-and-so's number." Once I've looked up the number (pretty easy), the behavioral ball is rolling, and I usually just go ahead and make the call. Psychologists call this *behavioral momentum*. I can't promise that this will always happen when you do a Task Chunk, but it can be a nice bonus.

You can also use:

❑ Timers (page 22)

To help you engage in a task, replace "I have to clean this WHOLE kitchen!" with "I have to work on cleaning the kitchen for 10 minutes." Then set the timer on your phone, oven, or microwave and get going. If you finish 10 minutes, great! If you keep going, even better.

Another strategy that can make task size more manageable and getting started less daunting is:

❑ The Pomodoro Technique (page 32)

This strategy involves breaking your task-related goals into smaller chunks of time, which can make things feel less overwhelming.

≫ C: I find myself doing everything *except* the thing I should be doing.

This is an incredibly frustrating situation, *but it actually contains a lot of useful information*. Specifically:

> *Whatever you're doing instead of the avoided task has the potential to be a reward for that task.***

---

*Truth be told, I'm enabled by my introverted but socially skilled husband who will, for example, call in our Chinese food orders.

I can't resist sharing that, in psychology, this idea is called the Premack principle. It means that rewards are not **things, but rather **activities**. It can be helpful to think about rewards this way because it expands the possible pool of things that might be rewarding.

"Instead" tasks are, surprisingly, not always super-enjoyable, maximally rewarding activities. Instead, they tend to just not be *as bad as* the avoided task. For example, when I was in college, at the end of each semester when I was supposed to be studying for finals, I suddenly had a deep and profound urge to clean and organize my dorm room. My own research has shown that when people are avoiding work tasks, they're most likely to be doing . . . other work tasks! So a rewarding activity need not be an all-out party—it just needs to be better than the alternative.

Reflect for a moment—when you are in "avoidance mode" for a hated task, what are you typically doing instead?

_____

_____

_____

To leverage this new information about what is (relatively) rewarding, you'll use these activities as rewards for completing some part of the avoided task. For example: "If I study chemistry for 30 minutes, I can organize my desktop." "If I grade two papers, I can refill my coffee." "If I finish writing this chapter, I can check my email."

To start using this strategy, review the section on:

❑ Rewarding Consequences (page 29)

Then you can combine the use of Rewarding Consequences with your Calendar System and try out some:

❑ Strategic Task Scheduling (page 31)

You could also use:

❑ Accountability Partners (page 33)

Accountability partners can provide additional Rewarding Consequences. A writing accountability group, for example, can provide cheerleading for getting started on a daunting task and provide empathic coaching when you need it.

>> **D: When I think about doing something I'm avoiding, I have a lot of negative thoughts, *or* I think things like "I'll have more time to do it later."**

We often avoid things because those things prompt thoughts and feelings that we want to escape. You feel anxious or overwhelmed by a task or just too tired, and so you think, "Actually, it's not a big deal if I do this later," and divert your attention elsewhere. But sooner or later the task looms again and the icky feelings are even worse.

It takes a lot of skill to recognize when this escape process is happening because it occurs so quickly and without awareness. Learning to respond differently to avoidance feelings is going to take some practice. Begin with:

❑ Choice Point Analysis (page 36)

Then practice new responses to these thoughts and feelings by diving into:

❑ Self-Coaching (page 40)

>> **E: I'm a human being, which means no matter what, sometimes I'm going to procrastinate.**

I am feeling this very deeply as I write this sentence. I'm not where I wanted to be in terms of progress on this book at the moment I'm writing this. I feel ashamed that I haven't made more progress at this point and that the deadline is so close. I didn't follow through on my timeline the way I said I would. Sure, there were lots of other competing priorities that I had across the past few months and some stressful things too, but . . . I'm supposed to be *the expert* on strategies to help with executive functioning struggles. And yet here I am. And this little voice whispers, "What right do YOU have to be giving yourself or anyone else advice on how to reduce procrastination?"

And even as I type this, I realize I'm at a choice point. This is an opportunity to practice what I preach and do some Self-Coaching. I can accept these negative thoughts and feelings as having some validity—I didn't meet the goals I wanted to hit, and it doesn't feel good. If I didn't care and writing this book wasn't meaningful or important to me, I wouldn't feel these feelings. My pain shows where my values are. *And* I have choices that are under my control and strategies I can use to move forward. First, I'm going to communicate with my editor and coauthor and apologize for not making more timely progress and ask to come up with a modified timeline. Next, I've been using strategies like the Pomodoro Technique and Accountability Partners, but I will also do more with Rewarding Consequences and Strategic Task Scheduling. And as for the Self-Coaching part, I'm going to read this paragraph again and then follow the steps I laid out. (And I guess if you're reading this, it all worked out!)

10

stick with it and wrap up

"If I could only figure out how to make boring tasks interesting, I could finally catch up on the paperwork sitting on my desk that I've been putting off for weeks."

Even if you're able to get started, you might have problems sticking with a task (after the novelty wears off) or wrapping up the final steps of a project, even when the goal is close at hand. The strategies in this chapter are designed to help you better understand the wrapping-up problems that might be getting in the way of your goals and to help you get unstuck.

Self-Assessment and Roadmap

Read each statement on the facing page and choose the best answer for you by putting a checkmark (✔) in the box. Use your answers to choose which sections to review.

- *A lot* like me!—Definitely review this section!

- Somewhat like me—Review this section if you need additional ideas.

- Not like me—This section doesn't seem to apply to you, so skip it if you want.

	Not like me	Somewhat like me	*A lot* like me!	Sections to review
I'm very easily distracted during boring tasks that require focus.				A (page 97)
I jump around from one task to another without finishing anything.				B (page 98)
I feel like everything I do has to be *just right* before wrapping up.				C (page 100)
I'm a human being, which means no matter what, I may struggle to stick with and finish things sometimes.				D (page 102)

» A: I'm very easily distracted during boring tasks that require focus.

First, you'll want to make sure you're setting yourself up for success by engineering a:

❑ Reduced-Distraction Environment (page 25)

Next, I recommend you check out:

❑ The Pomodoro Technique (page 32)

This technique can help you maximize your focus during bite-sized chunks of time. In particular, if you've stalled on a particular task and you've recognized that, committing to *even just* **one** *Pomodoro* (25 minutes) might help you make enough progress to generate some behavioral momentum and reduce your stuckness.

❑ Use an Accountability Partner (page 33).

This tool can also be very helpful to staying on task. For example, you could use body doubling—working in the presence of others in the physical world or online together—to help with follow-through.

≫ B: I jump around from one task to another without finishing anything.

Jumping from one task to another isn't *necessarily* a problem. Switching gears to a different way of using your brain when you're feeling burned out on a task can re-energize you and boost your motivation. But task switching too often can also be costly—especially if you have trouble getting back around to re-engage with the unfinished tasks. If you have unfinished projects all over your house, yard, or computer, this section is for you.

If you haven't already:

❑ Review the strategies listed under Section A above to help promote focus and possibly prevent too-frequent task switching.

Next, assess whether you're engaged with your:

❑ Task-Tracking System (page 17)

If not, your first step is going to be setting up this system, updating it, or otherwise re-engaging. Then ask yourself, "Are all my unfinished tasks somewhere in my Task-Tracking System?"

If not, it's time to do an inventory of your unfinished tasks. Grab a pen or pencil and first write down any tasks on the blanks below that you already know have been left hanging. Next, get ready to go on a tour! Literally walk around your house, garage, yard, car, and add to your inventory any unfinished tasks you discover.

Unfinished Task Inventory

_____	_____
_____	_____
_____	_____

How do you feel looking at your inventory? It might be overwhelming to come face to face with all the tasks that have fallen by the wayside. You're probably now at a choice point (page 36) where you could just keep ignoring these tasks (because focusing on them doesn't feel good) or choose to take a small step toward accomplishing these goals. In other words, it's time for some solid:

❑ Self-Coaching (page 40)

Include both encouragement and strategies in how you talk to yourself about this list—for example, "This list is long, and I feel tired and ashamed when I look at it. But this is the first step to addressing this problem, and I'm taking it right now, which is a thing to be proud of." This might also be a good time to get with an Accountability Partner (page 33) who can support your efforts. Next, you're going to get strategic about how to handle these unfinished tasks.

❑ For each item in the Unfinished Task Inventory, consider: *Is this task worth finishing?*

Life is full of choices about how to spend your time, and the fact that you've started a task doesn't mean you *must* finish it. We can often fall prey to the *sunk cost fallacy,* which leads us to irrationally continue to invest time, money, and energy when doing so is unlikely to benefit us. It can be emotionally hard to cut your losses and decide to give up on a goal, but sometimes this is the best choice, both practically and emotionally. Please *don't give up on a task that's truly important to you or potentially beneficial,* but:

❏ Give yourself permission to let go of unfinished tasks that no longer make sense for you.*

Remove these from your Unfinished Task Inventory. Now that you've focused your list on what's worthwhile to finish, use:

❏ Priority Labeling (or Sorting) (page 18)

This tool will help you decide where it will be most important to spend your time. Then add each task to your Task-Tracking System (page 17). Choose the most important task and use the strategies in Get Started and Restarted (Chapter 9, page 89) to move forward.

» C: I feel like everything I do has to be *just right* before wrapping up.

Sometimes people have trouble finishing things because of *perfectionism,* or the belief that something terrible will happen or they're a bad person if everything isn't the absolute best that it can be. People with ADHD may develop tendencies toward perfectionism in an effort to control their symptoms or prevent the kind of negative feedback they've received from people in the past. But sadly perfectionism can block you from actually achieving your goals—in other words, the perfect can be the enemy of the good and—more importantly—the complete.

If perfectionism is a serious problem for you, working through it might require resources beyond this book. I recommend the *CBT Workbook for Perfectionism* by Sharon Martin and *Thoughts and Feelings: Taking Control of Your Moods and Your Life* by McKay, Davis, and Fanning. Or speak with a mental health professional about how to work your way out of perfection paralysis.

In the meantime, here are a few strategies for beginning to loosen its hold:

---

*And clean up any materials related to the task *or* put this cleanup on your task list.

1. Perfectionism is a form of *all-or-nothing thinking,* or the irrational belief that (a) things fall into only categories of good/bad and (b) anything that isn't 100% good is therefore bad. Try writing down the thoughts you have when you feel stuck on a task and recognize when you might be locked into this erroneous mindset.

2. Underneath perfectionism there is often fear and anxiety. We avoid thinking deeply about our fears because doing so is scary, and so we never really think through what it is we're afraid of and consider whether it actually makes sense for us. Try this: Choose a task that you think you might be approaching with anxiety-motivated perfectionism. *What do you believe will happen* if you don't execute this task 100% perfectly? *What is your worst fear?*

_____

_____

_____

Reread what you wrote and answer the following questions:

How likely do you think it is that, if your work isn't perfect, this worst fear will actually happen? _____%

If this worst fear actually happened, what is the likelihood that you could *not* get through it? _____%

Now imagine that your best friend or your child was having the same anxious thoughts. What would you say to them, and how would you coach them through it?

_____

_____

_____

3. Next, reflect on what might count as *good enough* for the task you've been having trouble completing. Do you really have a clear idea about what's required? Maybe you need to talk to someone—like a boss or teacher—to find out what *good enough* is for this task or at least reread

the instructions. (You may have been overestimating what is required.) You could also seek feedback on your progress so far and ask questions to resolve your uncertainty.

Below, write some notes about what might be *good enough* for this task **or** some ideas about how you'll get information on this.

_____

_____

_____

Finally, go back and reread what you wrote for your worst fear in Step 2, then rerate:

How likely do you think it is that, if your work isn't perfect, this worst fear will actually happen? _____%

If this worst fear actually happened, what is the likelihood that you could *not* get through it? _____%

Did your ratings change? If not, that's okay—you can still focus on getting to good enough for your task. But changes in your ratings might suggest that anxious thoughts and feelings are just that— thoughts and feelings and not facts or things that **must** control your actions. Changing your perspective and focusing on actions can turn down the volume of your anxiety.

≫ D: I'm a human being, which means no matter what, I may struggle to stick with and finish things sometimes.

Problems with finishing things can be emotionally hard. The longer the task is unfinished, the heavier it feels and the more you might beat yourself up for not being able to wrap it up. But you've taken the first step by getting curious about the barriers to sealing the deal on important tasks—including taking stock of which tasks *are* still important. Congrats on taking the first step to getting unstuck.

11

switch gears when you need to

"I have episodes of hyperfocus symptoms related to my ADHD. Yet unlike some, I don't view it as a benefit. Yes, it's helped me dive deeply into some subjects I really wanted to specialize in—like making music, doing some writing, or coding. But I found that it can evolve into obsessions where I just can't use my executive function to stop what I'm doing until I'm completely exhausted. And it also causes me to miss other time-based tasks I really need to get done during the day. In that sense, it's a two-edged sword and needs to be managed."

Do you ever get into a state of *hyperfocus* where you're completely absorbed in an activity with little awareness of the passage of time? If so, you probably also know that it can be hard to deploy these hyperfocus states toward the most meaningful and important activities.

Self-Assessment and Roadmap

Read each statement on the next page and choose the best answer for you by putting a checkmark (✓) in the box. Use your answers to choose which sections to review.

- *A lot* like me!—Definitely review this section!
- Somewhat like me—Review this section if you need additional ideas.
- Not like me—This section doesn't seem to apply to you, so skip it if you want.

	Not like me	Somewhat like me	*A lot* like me!	Sections to review
Screen time sucks up hours of my day without leaving me much to show for it.				A (page 104)
I spend hours absorbed in a preferred activity and can't tell where the time went.				B (page 107)
I delay falling asleep until way later than I should.				C (page 108)
I'm a human being, which means no matter what, it can be hard to stop doing things I enjoy.				D (page 108)

》 A: Screen time sucks up hours of my day without leaving me much to show for it.

Extracting yourself from absorption in screen time is probably one of the most difficult self-control tasks to tackle, primarily because the corporations behind those screens have figured out exactly what to offer to you to hold your attention and convert it into money. To circumvent getting hooked on screens, you may have to learn to hack your digital environment to promote focus. First:

❑ Take stock of your current level of digital health by visiting *www.digitaldetox.com/score*.

This free quiz can give you a sense of where you stand in terms of the need to change your digital habits and possibly kick-start your motivation to make change. (I know it did for me.)

❑ Evaluate exactly where your digital time is going.

Which activities are your danger zones? Jot down the apps, sites, or activities that you think are taking up the most time and attention:

_____

Next, check the digital well-being section of your device settings for stats on your most frequent mobile phone activities. Write down any other apps or activities that are sucking up your time:

_____

Now you have a sense of which activities you'll need to address most.

❑ Explore digital well-being settings on your phone.

Both Android and Apple phones offer specific settings to help you limit and control screen time. I have an Android phone, which offers a section on digital well-being under Settings. Open the digital well-being settings on your phone and take a look. I was surprised by the number of options available, including:

- View stats for your screen time usage
- Set hourly or daily limits for each app on total screen time, notifications, and times opened
- Add a timer to the screen when using specific websites that "suck you in"
- Set up Bedtime or Focus mode: times during the night or day that the phone will go into grayscale, screen dark, and do not disturb modes

- Change notification settings for each app
- Add a widget to your home screen that displays your total screen time for the day; just click your home screen and hold, scroll down to digital well-being, and choose a spot to paste it

❑ Look at the list of time-sucking apps you made above and do one or more of the following:
  - Adjust the digital well-being settings to add a timer and add limits to problem apps.
  - Turn off notifications for problem apps, or at least turn off notifications for some events.
  - Move the icons for problem apps off your home screen, so they're harder to get to (an example of a Speed Bump, page 47).
  - Consider deleting problem apps from your phone altogether, and access those sites only through your phone's web browser.

❑ For problem use on your laptop or desktop, try the following:
  - Turn off or limit notifications from apps that steal your attention (in Settings).
  - Use web browser plug-ins like StayFocusd for Google Chrome to set limits on certain problem sites.
  - Use an app like Freedom, which allows you to set limits on *all* your devices using one program.

❑ Make and use a *phone jail*.

This is a specific place you'll put your phone before starting to focus (or sleep!). Designate a pocket in your work bag or backpack or create (and decorate if you want!) a small container where you will place your phone before you sit down to focus. You could even set up a reminder on the phone to pop up at scheduled work times: "Put me in jail!"*

---

*I envision a meme of Rich Uncle Pennybags from Monopoly peeking out from behind bars, like from a Get Out of Jail Free card.

» B: I spend hours absorbed in a preferred activity and can't tell where the time went.

These strategies are intended to help you either prevent unwanted hyperfocus or help you realize that it's happening so that you can direct your resources elsewhere.

❑ Investigate the strategies in Section A above on screen time, which might help you limit hyperfocus on digital activities.

❑ Use timers (page 22) to limit hyperfocus.

Before beginning an activity that usually "sucks you in," set a timer for the maximum amount of time you want to spend on that activity. The alarm going off will give you a moment to redirect yourself.

❑ Set a series of alarms (page 23) to sound while you focus on a difficult task.

When each alarm rings, mentally check whether you've fallen into misdirected hyperfocus. For example, you could set your phone and computer to deliver notifications each hour during the workday or while writing or studying that read something like "Are you focused on what matters?" When you see the notification, do a mental check as to whether it's time to refocus.

If these strategies don't seem to help you disengage from hyperfocus activities, it's time to do a:

❑ Choice Point Analysis (page 36) and Self-Coaching (page 40)

Direct your analysis and self-coaching toward those moments where you realize you should do something else but have thoughts like "I can just do this for a few more minutes" or "I'll just do this one thing before I stop."

» C: I delay falling asleep until way later than I should.

Because sleep is so important to brain health and because getting too little sleep can make ADHD symptoms even worse, I thought it was important to address this problem in the book. I'm not talking about times when you can't fall asleep even though you're sincerely trying to—I'm talking about times when you're doing something else but part of you knows you *should* be letting your body get some rest. My guess is that a lot of these times involve using screens in bed. You keep scrolling, scrolling, scrolling—even though your eyelids are heavy and you're not enjoying yourself anyway. If this is your problem, you can try the following:

- ❑ Set up bedtime settings (see Section A of this chapter) in your phone's digital wellness section.
- ❑ Remove the TV from your bedroom or make it a tablet-free zone.
- ❑ Make a phone jail (page 106) that's out of reach from your bed.

Choose a spot in the room that you can't reach from your bed and put your phone charger there (and only there). Make sure you get yourself an alarm clock, so you don't fall back into using your phone as your alarm clock and having it drift back to your bedside table.

- ❑ Use a Choice Point Analysis (page 36) to understand those moments when part of you knows you should go to bed— particularly if you notice thoughts like "I haven't done anything fun today, so I deserve to watch these videos." Then develop a Self-Coaching (page 40) response that emphasizes how good you'll feel after a good night's rest.

» D: I'm a human being, which means no matter what, it can be hard to stop doing things I enjoy.

It can be frustrating to wake up from hyperfocus and realize that you've lost far more time than you intended to a device or another activity that wasn't in line with your intentions. That lack of awareness is what makes this problem so hard to manage, so it's understandable that it happens. As you work toward managing your focus and bringing it in line with your intentions, do your best to remain patient with yourself and practice self-compassion. And, most importantly, celebrate even the small gains that you can make—10 minutes you spend on something you value versus something you don't might seem small, but 10-minute chunks add up over time, meaning that even small daily gains matter.

12

keep your commitments to others

"While I know what to do, as a person with ADHD, I may not always do what I know is best for me and the important people in my life. However, I won't give up."

Living well with ADHD is a matter of finding ways to define and live a personally meaningful life in the presence of the challenges that ADHD presents. For most people, cultivating connected and fulfilling relationships is a key part of living well. The challenges associated with ADHD can sometimes make it difficult to be who you want to be in relation to other people in your life—including being able to follow through on commitments you've made to others. This chapter pulls together strategies from throughout the book to help you make commitments thoughtfully and increase your chances of following through. You'll also get some ideas for what to do when—like every human—you don't live up to your aspirations.

Self-Assessment and Roadmap

Read each statement below and choose the best answer for you by putting a checkmark (✓) in the box. Use your answers to choose which sections to review.

- *A lot* like me!—Definitely review this section!
- Somewhat like me—Review this section if you need additional ideas.
- Not like me—This section doesn't seem to apply to you, so skip it if you want.

	Not like me	Somewhat like me	*A lot* like me!	Sections to review
I don't keep track of what I'm supposed to do and when.				A (page 111)
I take on too many commitments, become overwhelmed, and then can't follow through.				B (page 112)
I put off getting started on tasks.				C (page 114)
I have trouble sticking with or wrapping up tasks.				D (page 115)
I'm a human being, which means no matter what, sometimes I'll let others down.				E (page 115)

» A: I don't keep track of what I'm supposed to do and when.

Keeping your promises to others is going to require that you remember what those promises are and when you need to deliver on them, so commit or recommit to using a:

□ Calendar System (page 16)
□ Task-Tracking System (page 17)

❯❯ B: I take on too many commitments, become overwhelmed, and then can't follow through.

When people ask you to do something, it can feel good to say yes and bad to say no. You might overestimate your ability to accomplish all the tasks that you put on your plate and underestimate the size of the tasks you're taking on. Before we talk about strategies, let's get a more visceral understanding of the problem of overcommitment.

Imagine you're at a potluck—a dinner where each person brings a dish to share.* All available space on the long table is covered with luscious-looking homemade dishes. You're first in line. You grab a plate and notice that your host has purchased the flimsiest, single-ply, non-coated paper plates available—and you've got only one. Undaunted, you take a big scoop from the first dish on the table, followed by a spoonful of the second. As you go down the line, you notice that your plate is getting very full fast. The savory sauces from the casseroles are starting to soak into the plate. But you don't want to say no to any of these dishes! Besides, if someone sees that you don't take any of *their* dish, they'll be super upset with you . . . right? And there are people waiting behind you—you've got to keep moving. As you go down the line, your plate gets heavier and more moist, and your anxiety grows. You try to take smaller spoons of each dish, but it's not really help-ing—the plate feels like it's going to slip out of your hand. Finally, you're nearing the end of the line and you spot your *favorite food of all time!* "I can do it," you think. "I'm sure I have *just* enough room. I can do it *all!*" You attempt to gingerly place a portion of your favorite atop the other foods on your plate as carefully as possible, but the plate slips sideways out of your hand . . .

How does this story connect with the idea of overcommitment and your experience of it?

---

* In Central Pennsylvania where I grew up, this is known as a "covered dish supper."

_____

_____

_____

Here are a few things I think this story illustrates about over-commitment:*

- It can be hard to notice when it's happening because it happens little by little and, before you're aware of it, you can be overwhelmed.

- If can feel really good to say yes! Especially if you're a person who's generally concerned about pleasing others.

- Your plate doesn't have unlimited capacity. Overloading it creates stress.

- Taking on too much can limit your later opportunities for more meaningful things. Psychologists call this *opportunity cost*. In other words, saying yes to something now may mean having to say no to something else down the road.

Here are a few strategies to help you be more thoughtful in the commitments you make to others.

❑ Choose a default response you will give to requests that will buy time for you to consider them thoughtfully. This tip came from one of my grad school advisors, who suggested responding to any request for a commitment with:

That's really interesting. I'll have to think about that some more and get back to you.

This response gives you time to really weigh the pros and cons of the request and to avoid responding with an impulsive, people-pleasing

---

*I developed this story into a learning activity for some of my college students. They had to pile a flimsy paper plate with scoops of loose, melty Jell-O and walk, then run, across the lawn. The idea was to *feel* what it's like when you "put too much on your plate" and perhaps remember that feeling before taking on a new commitment. And when you have ADHD, you might need to be *even more* strategic about how much your plate can hold.

yes in the moment. An asker who is really motivated will follow up, even if you forget to.

❑ Ask for an estimated time commitment.

In addition to buying you time to consider, this question will give you information about the potential costs of a commitment. It may also reveal otherwise "hidden" aspects of the request—for example, the specific steps involved or how long the commitment will last.

❑ Ask yourself a series of key questions to help you reflect on whether you want to take on a commitment. Helpful questions to ask yourself include:

- Does taking on this commitment move me toward my personal values (see Chapter 26, page 197)?
- Is it likely that saying no will severely hurt my career or relationship?
- How will I feel when it comes time to actually do this task? (Will the You of the Future resent the You of Now for saying yes?)
- If I say yes to this, what other activities (or potential activities) will have to get less time and effort?
- What would I advise my best friend to do in this situation?

Best wishes in making these decisions! They are hard, but eliminating even a few less meaningful commitments from your plate can create space and reduce stress.

≫ C: I put off getting started on tasks.

Visit the strategies in:

❑ Get Started and Restarted (Chapter 9, page 89)

>> D: I have trouble sticking with or wrapping up tasks.

Visit the strategies in:

❏ Stick with It and Wrap Up (Chapter 10, page 96)

>> E: I'm a human being, which means no matter what, sometimes I'll let others down.

This is a tough one—especially if you have struggled with ADHD symptoms for a long time and they've impacted your ability to keep your promises to others. You might worry about what other people think of you and, even harder, might see *yourself* as a person who isn't worthy of others' trust. You may deeply mistrust yourself. If you feel like those two sentences really hit home, you're not alone and you might consider discussing these thoughts and feelings with a counselor or, better yet, a cognitive-behavioral therapist with experience in the ways that living with ADHD affects your self-beliefs (see the Resources, page 210). Dr. J. Russell Ramsay's book *Rethinking Adult ADHD* might be particularly helpful to you or your therapist. ADHD support groups (see Support Communities, page 52) can also give you access to people who can empathize with your experiences.

Despite how you feel, letting others down is something you are committing to working on just by reading this chapter. That's a big deal. And it's okay for you to ask others for patience and even help as you work toward getting better at fulfilling your commitments. It's okay to ask for reminders, for example—especially if you've agreed to do something for someone else. And if you do mess up, there are skillful ways to work toward repair. Read my recommendations for Effective Apologies (page 50) and engage with some constructive Self-Coaching (page 40) when you stumble in this (or any) area.

13

absorb information

"I can do things such as small tasks and not even realize it because my mind was elsewhere. I lose things, I misplace things, I don't listen well to what others are saying, and I make a lot of mistakes in my detail-oriented job. I get stuck in my head and disconnected from the world when I try to do anything I'm not interested in, including listening to others."

People with ADHD sometimes find they don't process or absorb information as quickly as other people. They may have to exert more willpower to stay focused on what they read or hear. If this is a challenge for you, read on.

Self-Assessment and Roadmap

Read each statement on the facing page and choose the best answer for you by putting a checkmark (✓) in the box. Use your answers to choose which sections to review.

- *A lot* like me!—Definitely review this section!
- Somewhat like me—Review this section if you need additional ideas.
- Not like me—This section doesn't seem to apply to you, so skip it if you want.

	Not like me	Somewhat like me	*A lot* like me!	Sections to review
I'm usually also on my phone or laptop or doing something else while trying to listen to or read something. (Be honest!)				A (page 117)
I have to read things over and over to get the meaning.				B (page 118)
I zone out when I'm trying to listen to lectures, meetings, or recordings.				C (page 120)
I have difficulty listening in conversations.				D (page 121)
I'm a human being, which means no matter what, I'm going to be slower at or struggle with some things more than others.				E (page 123)

≫ A: I'm usually also on my phone or laptop or doing something else while trying to listen to or read something. (Be honest!)

I'm not trying to tech-shame anyone, but attempts at mental *multitasking* are a major potential source of chronic difficulties with focusing on and absorbing information. Psychology research is clear: Humans cannot mentally multitask in the true sense of *actually being able to do two attention-demanding mental tasks at once.** Rather, what *appears* to be multitasking is really *switching of attention back and forth between two tasks.* This means that there will be loss of information for the task that's not

---

*You might be thinking "But I can drive a car and think about something else at the same time!" You may even be able to do other well-learned manual tasks like knitting while listening intently. Notice, however, that these "at the same time" tasks are physical tasks that are what psychologists call *overlearned*—that is, you've practiced and practiced them so that the work has been transferred to a different part of your brain, and those programs can run without much active attention—that is, **until** something unexpected happens (a car pulls out; you notice you missed a stitch). When it comes to, for example, listening to and comprehending a lecture and shopping on Amazon, your brain can't do both at once.

currently in the spotlight of attention. For people with ADHD, task switching may be even more costly than for others.

Because I'm a professor, I'm particularly familiar with the research on use of distracting technology in the college classroom. The results are consistent, and they're not pretty. Students who are struggling the most are also the ones hurt the most by the presence of distracting tech in the classroom. Even students sitting *near* the person using their laptop to multitask during lectures get lower grades due to second-hand distraction. The research is so clear that I strongly encourage my students not to use laptops in class unless we're using them for a class activity.

So if you're trying to pay attention and truly comprehend the information being communicated, first remove or regulate your use of screens in those situations. To do so, visit Section A in:

❑ Switch Gears When You Need To (Chapter 11): Screen time sucks up hours of my day without leaving me much to show for it (page 104)

❯❯ B: I have to read things over and over to get the meaning.

Adults with ADHD that I've worked with over the years have often struggled with trying to read complicated texts. They zone out halfway down the page and then have to reread to get the information. This can make completing reading assignments frustrating and inefficient, to say the least. If that sounds like you, here are some strategies to try.

Sometimes reading difficulties arise when you're trying to "cram" or push your attention up against its limits. To provide adequate breaks to replenish your reading resources, use:

❑ The Pomodoro Technique (page 32)

Pomodoro provides built-in breaks that can also serve as check-ins as to whether you're still focused. Although a Pomodoro is traditionally 25 minutes long, you can shorten that time period if you need to do deep reading of dense texts.

Some people find it easier to pay attention to spoken text—this is certainly the case for me. You could also read and listen simultaneously to boost focus. Fortunately, screen-reading technology has gotten better, cheaper, and more accessible than ever. So you could:

❑ Use screen reading on your phone or computer instead of (only) reading with your eyes.

For example, on my PC under Settings → Ease of Access there is a section called Narrator that allows me to turn on screen reading and to customize how it works. This is a great example of how making environments more accessible for people with certain disabilities (in this case, people with vision problems) provides resources for others. Thanks, inclusion!

Finally, you can use some tried-and-true strategies from the science of reading to boost comprehension of information-packed texts like textbook chapters, articles, and professional documents. These documents can be hard to read "straight through" and actually absorb. One of the most well known is a set of five strategies called *SQ3R,* which stands for:

❑ Survey, question, read, recite, review (SQ3R)

Virginia Tech has an excellent website describing the components of SQ3R at *https://ucc.vt.edu/academic_support/study_skills_information/ sq3r_reading-study_system.html* if you want to learn more. Briefly, the SQ3R steps are:

- First, **survey** the text by reading just the title, introduction, headings, graphics, and any in-text summaries. This helps you develop a framework for what you'll read.

- Use your survey of the text, especially the headings, to develop **questions** that you think the text will answer. Write down these questions so you can remember them. As you read, you will be searching for the answers to these questions. This can help you zero in on the most important information and keep you engaged in the hunt while reading.

- **Read** the text a section a time and write down the answers you find to the questions you wrote down.

- At the end of each section, **recite**—or test yourself—on the answers to each question to boost your memory.

- After you complete the entire reading, **review** everything by quizzing yourself again on the answers to all the questions.

This probably sounds like a lot, but even trying to incorporate the survey/question/read steps of the process just might boost your engagement with the text enough to reduce problems with zoning out. Give it a shot!

If problems with reading speed, accuracy, and comprehension persist, it may be a good idea to:

❑ Consider a clinical assessment, including testing for learning differences (see the Resources, page 209).

People with ADHD are more likely than those without ADHD to be diagnosed with learning disorders, including reading disorders.* But these disorders sometimes go undiagnosed when people use other strengths to compensate for reading problems. A professional assessment can clarify the issue.

» C: I zone out when I'm trying to listen to lectures, meetings, or recordings.

One way to reduce zoning out is to engage more actively with what you're listening to by:

❑ Taking notes as you listen—preferably by hand

Most people think about taking notes just so they can look back at them later. But lots of research shows that taking notes while

---

* *Dyslexia* is another word for a reading disorder. Although many people think dyslexia only refers to "reversing letters," there are many more varieties of dyslexia (reading disorder) that can be diagnosed by educational psychologists.

listening—especially by hand—increases focus and memory, even if you never look at the notes you create. So consider note taking a tool that could focus you.

Can you, like some people with ADHD, focus better when your hands are occupied or other parts of your body are moving? If so, you could:

❑ Use fidget toys or other physical tasks that are "automatic" for you while listening.

For example, I know people who can listen and focus better while simultaneously knitting. Importantly, these are *experienced* knitters whose hands knit relatively automatically without pulling away their attention from listening.* So if you're going to try this, choose something you really can do automatically without devoting much attention to it. Don't try to learn a new skill for this purpose. Also, it's a good idea to explain to the people you're listening to how doing this other task helps you listen. Otherwise it could be distracting (and maybe demoralizing!) to a speaker who isn't aware of why you're doing something else while they're talking.

If you are trying to pay attention to a recording:

❑ Turn on closed captioning for video or audio recordings.

For example, most YouTube videos have captions you can turn on. My Android phone has a Live Caption feature that allows me to see captions on, for example, my favorite podcasts. Taking in information through more than one sense simultaneously could help improve focus.

» D: I have difficulty listening in conversations.

Conversations—especially long ones—can be an attention challenge for people with ADHD. You might find yourself zoning out or interrupting because it's difficult to wait to get your point across. There

---

*If you're thinking: "Wait, I thought you said people can't actually multitask!" please read the footnote on page 117.

are lots of tips out there on *active listening,* which is an idea originally developed by psychotherapists to describe how to fully engage with clients and help them feel heard and validated. Active listening strategies focus on the idea of *listening to understand* instead of *listening to respond.* Specific recommendations include *putting away any devices* and periodically *reflecting back or summarizing* what the person has said to check your understanding.

While active listening strategies can be helpful, I'm not sure they are always the most applicable to a two-way conversation, which involves functioning as both the listener and the speaker. In conducting research for this book, I happened upon a wonderful TED Talk by professional interviewer Celeste Headlee that emphasizes an important point. She said the key to good listening and, by extension, good conversation is to:

❏ Cultivate genuine curiosity about the people you talk to.

As Headlee describes it, "Everyone is an expert in something," and assuming that you have something to learn from every conversation can help you stay focused on what's being said. For people with ADHD, interest drives attention, and so increasing your interest in others and practicing a few strategies to get more interesting responses from people—such as asking only open-ended questions—could improve your conversations.

I recommend you check out Headlee's talk at *https://youtu.be/ R1vskiVDwl4* and jot down a couple of strategies you want to try. And if you want to go deeper, check out *The Lost Art of Listening* by Michael P. Nichols, PhD, and Martha B. Straus, PhD.

Finally, if your brain is more engaged by images than words, you could try to:

❏ Build a visual image of what a person is saying to you as you listen.

Consider a mental concept map or a visualization of the story they're telling you. This might help boost focus and help you follow the story.

》 E: I'm a human being, which means no matter what, I'm going to be slower at or struggle with some things more than others.

Even if you find some strategies that help you, you might process information more slowly than other people or struggle to maintain focus. This can be difficult to accept—to feel like you're falling behind or always playing a game of catch-up compared to others. It's true that everyone has strengths and weaknesses, but knowing that fact doesn't necessarily make coping with *your* weaknesses any easier. It can be hard not to compare yourself to other people. But some of the best advice I've gotten on this is to *stay in your lane*. In other words, you're running your own race at your own pace toward your goals. You've striving to live a little bit better with your ADHD than you did yesterday or last week or last year. That might mean you take longer to reach certain goals than others or do so having to navigate more struggles, making it even more important to *celebrate even small wins*. You'll be giving yourself motivational fuel to move forward.

14

manage restlessness

"I figured out a long time ago that to do a desk job I needed to work out really intensively almost daily. And luckily I've been able to set up my office so that I can stand and pace around when I need to. But sometimes it still feels uncomfortable to just have to SIT and I dread it."

People with ADHD sometimes struggle with feelings of internal restlessness or discomfort—especially in less stimulating situations. Importantly, this sense of restlessness is somewhat different than restlessness that's associated with anxiety, so it's important to know that this chapter doesn't address anxiety-related restlessness.

Self-Assessment and Roadmap

Read each statement on the facing page and choose the best answer for you by putting a checkmark (✓) in the box. Use your answers to choose which sections to review.

- *A lot* like me!—Definitely review this section!
- Somewhat like me—Review this section if you need additional ideas.
- Not like me—This section doesn't seem to apply to you, so skip it if you want.

	Not like me	Somewhat like me	*A lot* like me!	Sections to review
I can't sit for long periods of time without feeling distractingly uncomfortable.				A (page 125)
I experience overwhelming urges to escape a tedious or frustrating task or situation.				B (page 127)
I get so exhausted having to monitor my behavior all the time and use all these tools to keep myself in check.				C (page 128)

» A: I can't sit for long periods of time without feeling distractingly uncomfortable.

If you have a job that involves a lot of physical movement, this might not be too much of a problem for you. In an office setting, you might try to avoid sitting for long periods of time as much as you can. Fortunately, many workplaces are a little less formal than they used to be in terms of demanding that people remain seated at their desks for 8 hours a day.

❑ Schedule movement breaks throughout the day.

Put these in your Calendar System (page 16). Take a lap around the office or your house or, better yet, outside around the building or the block. If you're using the Pomodoro Technique (page 32), make sure your 5-minute breaks involve movement. If long meetings are a problem, request a pause every 30 minutes for the group to gather its collective thoughts and move around if needed.

Another creative solution is to:

❑ Use a standing desk.

Standing desks are more popular than ever, and though there are fancy and pricey versions out there, they don't have to be expensive. My husband made himself a standing desk out of old file cabinets and a board. Standing desks are great because they allow you to engage more easily in movement while trying to focus. If you need to both sit and stand, there are adjustable desk options as well.

Sometimes people with ADHD report that they're able to focus better when their hands are occupied or other parts of their body are moving. In the autism community this is known as *stimming*—a coping strategy people might use to help regulate emotions, sensations, or focus. In my opinion, we shouldn't overpathologize fidgeting and stimming that doesn't cause a person any substantial problems.* Fortunately, more clinicians and members of the public are taking this perspective, inspired by neurodiverse people themselves. So:

❑ If you have to sit for a long time, use fidget toys or engage in physical tasks that are "automatic" for you.

The array of fidget toys and devices available these days is quite diverse, so try out a few and see what works best for you. As mentioned in Chapter 13 (page 121), some people can focus while simultaneously knitting. Importantly, these are *experienced* knitters whose hands can knit relatively automatically without pulling away their attention from listening. If there's a skill you have that fits this category, you could try that. If you're fidgeting or knitting or whatever is noticeable, it's a good idea to explain to the people around you how fidgeting helps you focus so that they understand the purpose of it. You'll also be helping reduce stigma for other stimmers!

Finally, over the years I have met many people with ADHD who say that regular, vigorous physical exercise is absolutely essential for them to stay focused for the rest of the day. If this applies to you:

---

*In this case I'm definitely not talking about stimming that causes harm to autistic people, such as head banging or other behaviors that result in self-injury.

❑ Schedule regular exercise times in your Calendar System (page 16) and fiercely protect them.

Show yourself as unavailable at that time in your work calendar. Exercise is not a luxury—it's a responsibility you have to others and to yourself to be able to function at your best.

❯❯ B: I experience overwhelming urges to escape a tedious or frustrating task or situation.

Many adults with ADHD describe moments when, emotionally, they can't tolerate staying still or continuing to engage with a task—usually one that's boring, frustrating, or tedious. From what people describe to me, this seems to go beyond run-of-the-mill boredom and seems more like an emotional urge that is very hard to resist. Examples of situations that can induce these urges include waiting in line, filling out forms, or being trapped in tedious conversation.

Like any urge, there are ways to manage these feelings and to reduce their negative consequences. For example, while waiting, you can engage in:

❑ A time crack task (page 61) to occupy your mind or body.
❑ Fidgeting or stimming.

If you must:

❑ Take a break from the task or situation—especially one that involves movement.
❑ Make sure the unfinished task is in your Task-Tracking System (page 17) with a note about exactly where you left off.

To manage these urges and try to calm your emotions in the moment and re-engage, you can also use:

❑ Your personal Emotional Antidotes (page 46)

» C: I get so exhausted having to monitor my behavior all the time and use all these tools to keep myself in check.

This struggle is real, and there's a good reason for it. Self-regulation requires energy, and, for people with ADHD, engaging willpower might deplete energy reserves faster than for others. Even as you're working toward your goals, think of living well with ADHD as a marathon, not a sprint. *You will need to take self-regulation and restoration breaks, and that is more than okay.*

What's most restorative varies from person to person, so it's a good idea to get curious about what kinds of activities fill up your personal self-regulation bucket the most. Jot down some ideas below.

Write down three activities that you don't have to force yourself to do that leave you feeling the most restored.

_____

_____

_____

I could be wrong, but my guess is that "scrolling mindlessly on Reddit" or "binge watching crappy true crime shows" might be unlikely to show up on your personal restoration list.* These activities wouldn't show up on mine either, and yet *these are the sorts of things I find myself doing in my "free time"* rather than truly restorative activities like listening to my Nina Simone record collection, playing Jackbox Games with my family, or sitting outside under the stars at night. It just doesn't occur to me to do things when I'm feeling tired and depleted. How about you?

If you're like me, I'm going to encourage you to:

❑ Develop a Restorative Fun Menu.

This is simply a list of enjoyable and restorative activities. You can start with the three things you wrote above and then brainstorm more.

---

*In a recent study my lab conducted, we found that when people were avoiding household chores, they were often engaging in screen time instead.

Ideas for good menu items include creative hobbies that provide a sense of accomplishment and engagement with the sensory world such as arts, crafts, dance, sports and games, cooking, or learning and playing music. Then:

❑ Post your Restorative Fun Menu somewhere you'll see it often.

Then, when you find yourself with some free time, it'll be easier to think of these ways to spend your time. Better yet:

❑ Schedule restorative fun in your Calendar System (page 16) and protect it fiercely.

If you're struggling to fill your menu with items, check out this list of 365 potentially pleasurable activities, the *Fun Activities Catalogue,* offered by the Centre for Clinical Interventions in Western Australia: *https://cci.health.wa.gov.au/-/media/CCI/Mental-Health-Professionals/ Depression/Depression---Information-Sheets/Depression-Information-Sheet- --06---Fun-Activities-Catalogue.pdf.*

15

manage the urge to act out when you're upset

"I am VERY patient until I'm not. It's like I have no middle ground here. Over the years I have learned to be 'kinder' when my emotions overflow, but it's still a very surprising thing for people I am with. I know I have this problem, so it's not a lack of awareness but difficulties with down-regulating strong feelings can really impact my relationships."

Although it's not part of the "official" diagnosis, most adults with ADHD report difficulties related to strong emotions—especially negative emotions—and the way they react to situations that provoke these emotions. Maybe you find that you're quicker than most people to become irritable, impatient, or upset in response to the delays and hassles of daily life (traffic jams, long lines, and frozen computer screens). Or perhaps what you've said and done in anger has damaged your relationships with other people and kept you from being the person you want to be with those you love. Maybe once you are upset it's very hard for you to calm yourself and see the situation from any alternative perspectives.

It doesn't *feel* good to experience these strong negative reactions, and you may have found that this emotional impulsivity seems difficult to control and hard to change. If so, you are not alone and it's not too surprising. Emotions evolved to motivate us to act, and they are a full body and mind response, influencing what we feel physically, how our minds focus and filter our experiences, and the kinds of reactions we have. But fortunately we also know that people can use strategies to manage and modify their emotional experiences and to channel emotions in more constructive ways.

To identify which strategies might be the most helpful for you, complete the self-assessment that follows. Because of the powerful effect of emotions on actions and the impact of ADHD on this process, emotional impulsivity can be among the most difficult patterns for adults with ADHD to change on their own. As always, if the ideas in this chapter seem potentially helpful but you just can't seem to implement them consistently on your own, you might benefit from working with a cognitive-behavioral therapist (see the Resources) who can support your efforts.

Self-Assessment and Roadmap

Read each statement on the next page and choose the best answer for you by putting a checkmark (✓) in the box. Use your answers to choose which sections to review.

- *A lot* like me!—Definitely review this section!

- Somewhat like me—Review this section if you need additional ideas.

- Not like me—This section doesn't seem to apply to you, so skip it if you want.

	Not like me	Somewhat like me	*A lot* like me!	Sections to review
In specific "trigger" situations, I get upset quickly and act out.				A (page 132)
Once I'm upset, it's really hard for me to calm my body.				B (page 134)
When I'm upset, I can't seem to focus my mind on anything else.				C (page 135)
When I'm upset, it's hard to see the situation in a way that's *not* upsetting.				D (page 136)
I'm a human being, which means no matter what, at times I'm going to say and do things I later regret.				E (page 139)

» A: In specific "trigger" situations, I get upset quickly and act out.

Try making a list of your impulsive emotion danger zones and your responses. Think about the times when your strong emotional responses have caused the most problems for you or your relationships. Maybe it's a conversation with a particularly challenging family member or having to call customer service *again* or passing that slow driver who refuses to move over to the right lane.

Write down your top three danger zones and your less-than-ideal responses:

1. When _____, I _____.
2. When _____, I _____.
3. When _____, I _____.

You're going to work with this situation in two ways:

1. Identify ways you can minimize contact with these situations or prep yourself for them.
2. Identify ways you can put Speed Bumps (page 47) between you and impulsive actions.

First, for each situation, think of a way you could:

❑ Reduce contact with the situation and/or
❑ Enter the situation when you're better emotionally prepared

For example, if telephone conversations with a particular family member usually result in a shouting match, you could choose to communicate via email instead. You could schedule your telephone conversations with this family member in your calendar rather than answering the phone "on the fly" when you might be stressed out or distracted.

For each danger zone you wrote down, write down a strategy you could use to limit exposure to the situation or control the circumstances so that you're more emotionally prepared.

1. _____

2. _____

3. _____

Next, we're going to look at the space between the situation and your response to it and try to put some distance in there.

❑ Insert Speed Bumps (page 47) to delay your response.

A Speed Bump *could* be as simple as the classic "count to 10" rule, but I'd like to encourage you to get more creative. For example, if my problem response is to dash off a snarky email to my family member, I can set up a rule in my email system that will delay the sending of any email I send to that person for the length of time I specify. Then I have the chance to recall the email when I cool down a little.

Below, write out some Speed Bump ideas for any of the situations you identified above.

_____

_____

_____

» B: Once I'm upset, it's really hard for me to calm my body.

Emotions are not "all in your head." Instead, your whole body responds when you experience an emotion—especially strong, negative emotions. To give your body the best chance to calm down when you experience a strong emotion like anger, do what you can to:

❑ Leave the situation if at all possible.

This can be particularly hard to do if you're feeling angry because anger is an "approach" emotion that motivates you to act. Sometimes the wisest thing you can do is to remove yourself from the situation—not permanently, necessarily, but long enough for your body and mind to regulate itself.

For example, if you experience "road rage," your instinct in the moment will be to engage with whatever person you think has wronged you. Instead, acting the opposite—that is, pulling over and disengaging—might prevent an accident or other consequence you might later regret.

If for some reason you're unable to exit the situation, you may need to:

❑ Insert Speed Bumps (page 47) to delay your response.

For example, if you can feel yourself becoming angry and frustrated during a meeting, you can unobtrusively set a timer on your phone for 3 minutes and delay responding to the discussion until that time is up. Even take a bathroom break if you can. During that time, you could use tried-and-true deep breathing or other:

❑ Moments of Mindfulness (page 44)

These will be especially helpful if they're ones you've practiced *before* the challenging situation.

≫ C: When I'm upset, I can't seem to focus my mind on anything else.

Emotions don't just live in the body; they also change the way your brain processes information. Strong emotions—especially negative ones—can focus your attention and memory on things that reinforce and intensify those emotions. That's why an argument tends to prompt you to think of all the *other* times the person has irritated you, which can feed into your current frustrated state. How can you try to broaden and refocus your attentional lens?

Again, it might be a good idea to:

❑ Leave the situation if possible.

Give your brain a chance to reset (see above in Section B). While you're taking a break, it might be a good time to:

❑ Use an Emotional Antidote (page 46).

Refocusing your attention on an experience that's incompatible with your strong negative emotion might help turn down the volume. Humor, in particular, has a way of turning our perspective on its head—in a good way—when we're taking ourselves or the situation too seriously.

Speaking of attention and perspective, remember that mindfulness is all about paying attention on purpose without judgment. So perhaps redirecting your attention toward something other than the triggering irritation could be useful. Try using a:

❑ Moment of Mindfulness (page 44)

Remember, however, that if you're trying any of these strategies, you may need to wait, wait . . . and then wait some more until your body and brain are ready to re-engage. That can be *very hard* when you're revved up, so if chronic acting out is a problem for you, it might be helpful to have an:

❑ Accountability Partner (page 33)

Someone who knows your struggles might help coach you through it when you're upset.

» D: When I'm upset, it's hard to see the situation in a way that's *not* upsetting.

When you're upset, it can feel like there is only one possible (upsetting) explanation for the situation that has upset you. Strong emotions not only affect what you pay attention to and what comes to mind; they influence your interpretation of the meaning of people's words and actions. When getting angry at someone, you're more likely to assume that their actions were *intentional* and *personally directed toward you*. Then this interpretation stokes your negative feelings.

For example, imagine you're driving along minding your own business and someone cuts you off so that you have to hit your brakes to avoid a collision. Most people probably *don't* instinctively think "Ah, well, I bet that person is worried about something stressful in their life and they just didn't notice. I wish them well!" (Okay, maybe you do, but if so you're a better person than I am.) Instead, most people probably instantaneously think something like "What the ****! Why are you being a jerk to me?" and might even think it's time for getting even. And yet, my guess is *we've all been that person who has cut someone off accidentally* at some point. Our brains just aren't good at considering that alternative possibility—especially in stressful situations that require high alert, like driving. So thinking more flexibly is probably going to take some practice.

A helpful strategy is to:

> Recognize the story you're telling yourself
> about the situation.

Rarely do any of us have 100% of the facts about any situation. Our emotional brains are going to fill in the blanks. And we can feel **so sure** that the story we're telling ourselves is accurate! This reminds me of one of my favorite things on the internet—a video of a commencement speech by the late David Foster Wallace entitled "This Is Water" (*https://youtu.be/eC7xzavzEKY*). In the speech Wallace talks about getting unstuck from our *default setting,* which is to make uncharitable assumptions about other's people behavior and to interpret their actions as intentional and personal. And then these default setting interpretations feed our annoyance and frustration instead of broadening our sense of a shared humanity. But I'm not doing it justice—please check it out!

Back to the task at hand. Labeling your thoughts about a situation as a *story,* which may or may not be true, can help you step back and take stock of where you might be jumping to conclusions versus where you might be having genuine insights.

Let's practice. Think of a recent situation where another person did something that you got upset about. Write down what the person did below. **Note:** *Do not write any interpretations, evaluations, or labels.* Just the facts of their words or actions that people other than you could also have observed.

_____

_____

_____

On a scale of 1–10 (10 being the most), how upset do you feel about the situation now? _____

Now ask yourself: *What is the story I'm telling myself* about these actions? Include your assumptions about why the person did this and what their intentions were.

_____

_____

_____

> **Important before we proceed:** I am not saying that this person's actions might not have been harmful, unjust, or immoral. I'm only asking you to examine your thinking about them.

Reread what you wrote and answer the following questions:

Were you making any assumptions about the causes of this person's actions? If so, what are alternative or additional explanations?

_____

_____

_____

Were you making any assumptions about this person's intent or purpose in taking these actions? If so, what are alternative or additional explanations?

_____

_____

_____

On a scale of 1–10 (10 being the most), how upset do you feel about the situation now? _____

Did you notice anything interesting? Did your emotional intensity change? Maybe, maybe not. Hopefully, either way, this was good practice for being able to step back from the stories you may be telling yourself when you're upset. This re-evaluation can help you make wiser choices about how to respond.

Finally, think about how you can skillfully respond in situations like this. Is there anything you would like to do about this specific situation to resolve any remaining issues or prevent difficulties in the future? For example, you could use Clear Requests from the Toolbox (page 48) to express your perspective and ask the person to respond differently in the future. Any other ideas?

_____

_____

_____

Remember, thoughts and feelings are just that—not facts or things that must control your actions. Changing your perspective and focusing on strategies to improve the situation can turn down the volume on your anger and frustration. If you want to practice using the strategy of *recognizing the story you're telling yourself,* you can incorporate it into:

❑ Self-Coaching (page 40)

Finally, if you want to go deeper with the skills in this chapter, especially if anger remains a problem for you, check out *The Anger Management Workbook* by W. Robert Nay, PhD.

≫ E: I'm a human being, which means no matter what, at times I'm going to say and do things I later regret.

It can be painful to acknowledge the times that we've said or done things that we regret—things that may have harmed others. Our automatic response might be to dismiss, minimize, or otherwise avoid thinking about it. But if we do that, we miss the opportunity to do better in the future, to be the people we want to be, and to make repairs where we can. If the time is right, review Effective Apologies (page 50) and consider taking that step. It won't be easy, but it will probably be worth it.

16

make thoughtful decisions

"I'm a social guy and I really like helping people and making them happy, but it means that I'm often promising more than I can deliver. I'm also an optimist, and it'll all work out, but sometimes that means I get myself into trouble when it comes to decisions."

Acting on impulse is something that many—but not all—adults with ADHD struggle with. It makes sense that managing impulsivity is difficult, given that preventing impulsive actions first requires you to *stop*, but *stopping* is exactly the problem. For that reason, learning to make decisions more thoughtfully instead of on impulse will involve spending some time figuring out when you're most vulnerable to impulsive decisions and then setting up and, most importantly, practicing strategies for slowing down in those situations.

You'll notice that the descriptions of impulsive decisions in this chapter emphasize decisions made when you're feeling positive emotions. Of course, negative emotions can motivate impulsive behavior too. For additional strategies specific to negative emotions, see Chapter 15 (page 130).

Self-Assessment and Roadmap

To focus your efforts in this section, check off the area of decision making you *most want to work on:*

❑ Spending money

❑ Getting involved in business ventures

❑ Making commitments or promises you can't keep

❑ Using substances

❑ Having risky sex

❑ Other risky behavior: _____

❑ Other: _____

Next, read each statement below and on the next page and choose the best answer for you by putting a checkmark (✓) in the box. Use your answers to choose which sections to review.

- *A lot* like me!—Definitely review this section!

- Somewhat like me—Review this section if you need additional ideas.

- Not like me—This section doesn't seem to apply to you, so skip it if you want.

	Not like me	Somewhat like me	*A lot* like me!	Sections to review
I act based on what feels good or right in the moment, and then it gets me in trouble.				A (page 142)
I probably say yes more than I should just to please other people.				B (page 145)

	Not like me	Somewhat like me	*A lot* like me!	Sections to review
I tend to be overly optimistic about how things will turn out and overlook the downsides.				C (page 145)
I'm a human being, which means no matter what, I'm going to make the wrong decision sometimes.				D (page 148)

≫ A: I act based on what feels good or right in the moment, and then it gets me in trouble.

I'm not trying to be a downer here—often it's an *amazing* thing to act on good feelings in the moment! But if you're reading this, you're acknowledging that these kinds of decisions can get you into trouble. So for the problem area you checked off on the previous page, commit to the following rule:

> *When it comes to* _____, *I will act based on a plan, not a feeling.*

Repeat this to yourself a few times.

What should your plan look like? There are at least three steps to formulating your plan:

1. What is your goal?
2. What are the barriers to hitting this goal?
3. What is the plan to address those barriers?

For example, if your problem area is spending money impulsively on eating out and takeout, your plan might look like this:

> Goal: I want to stick to spending no more than $100 per month on eating out and takeout.

Barriers: Keeping track of the $100. Feeling too tired to cook. Friends inviting me out for dinner.

Plan for barriers:

- I'll put $100 into my Venmo from checking at the start of the month for eating out.
- I'll cook meals for the week on Sunday afternoons (which I enjoy) and also have some cheap, ready-to-heat meals on hand.
- I'll let my good friends know about my eating-out budgeting goal and suggest cheaper places to eat or other activities like going to the park or having them over for a movie and microwave popcorn.

Let's practice developing one of these plans.

Goal: For your problem area, what is a *specific* and *reasonable* goal to start with?

_____

_____

_____

Now reread your goal. Is it specific enough so that you'll know when you've accomplished it? For example, "spend less money on going out to eat" is too vague because how much less is enough to count? $10? $1? For goals, specific is always better. Revise your goal if needed.

Barriers: What's going to get in the way of meeting your goal? Where do you think you'll go off track?

_____

_____

_____

Important: You might not (yet) know what all the barriers are! And that's okay—you're just getting started. The truth is that *you probably won't know what all the barriers are until one of them causes your plan to fail!* This is to be expected, and it's a chance to make your plan even better—though it can be hard to look at it that way when your plans go off track. Another good tool to identify barriers is a Choice Point Analysis (page 36), which will help you identify the situations, thoughts, and feelings that might be important to address in your plan.

Plan 1.0: Based on your goal and your guesses about barriers, write out the steps you'll take and the tools you'll use to enact your plan. Toolbox tools that could be especially helpful parts of your plan include:

- Alarms, Reminders, and Prompts (page 23)
- Rewarding Consequences (page 29)
- Strategic Task Scheduling (page 31)
- Accountability Partners (page 33)
- Self-Coaching (page 40)
- Emotional Antidotes (page 46)
- Speed Bumps (page 47)

_____

_____

_____

_____

If this turned into more than a practice exercise and you feel ready, take the steps to enact your plan. Expect that you'll need to modify it as you go. If modifications are needed, make your Plan 2.0.

» B: I probably say yes more than I should just to please other people.

Refer to the strategies in Section B of Keep Your Commitments to Others (Chapter 12, page 112).

» C: I tend to be overly optimistic about how things will turn out and overlook the downsides.

Even if you've developed a plan for specific problem areas, life is going to present you with decisions that you don't plan for. Sometimes people with ADHD run into trouble because they may be overly optimistic about these decisions—seeing the possible upsides and either missing or downplaying the possible costs and consequences. It's true that there are lots of psychological benefits to a generally optimistic outlook on life, and I'm *not* here to "yuck your yum" when it comes to having a hopeful perspective. But because you've indicted some awareness that you might tend to be overly optimistic, following are some strategies for more balanced decision making.

To practice, choose a "yes/no" decision you made recently or one that you'll be making in the near future. If you can't think of anything, just make up an example.

Deciding whether or not to: _____.

- ❑ Next, fill in the chart on the next page with the pros and cons of doing and not doing this thing.
- ❑ Finally, give each pro or con a rating, 1–10, based on how pro-y or con-y each of them is.

Note: I don't recommend just adding up your scores to figure out what decision to make. The point of the number labeling is just to help you reflect on how important each reason is to you.

On page 147 is an example of what I might have written when deciding whether to write this book.

DECISION-MAKING PROS AND CONS

	Pros	Cons
Doing the thing		
Not doing the thing		

	Pros	Cons
Doing the thing (writing the book)	Helping more people with ADHD—10 Looks good on résumé—3 Book royalties—2 Can be creative—8 Satisfying to use my expertise—5	Time consuming—8 More stress/anxiety/pressure—8 Worry that it won't be any good—2
Not doing the thing (Not writing the book)	More time for other projects—5 More time with family—10 Avoid stress/anxiety—1	Miss opportunity to do something in line with my values—4 Might not have another opportunity like this again—4

How does this exercise help? First, it forces you to think about both the pros and the cons of a particular course of action. Second, asking you to reflect on the consequences of **not** choosing to do a particular thing can reveal *opportunity costs,* or hidden consequences of saying yes to something that will take up time you won't be able to devote to other pursuits. Finally, the importance ratings help you reflect on your own values. You can use this technique anytime you want to slow your roll and consider a decision in a more balanced way (the blank form is available to download and print at *www.guilford.com/knouse-materials*).

Decision making is also a very wise time to employ:

❑ Accountability Partners (page 33) and Support Communities (page 52)

People in your life can be a great sounding board for talking through your decision and helping you see it from more angles. You can even play devil's advocate and practice arguing in favor of the choice you're leaning away from, which can also provide perspective.

**>> D: I'm a human being, which means no matter what, I'm going
to make the wrong decision sometimes.**

Even if you're the wisest person in the world, you're going to make
decisions that don't turn out the way you planned. This can bring up
especially difficult feelings if in retrospect you recognize that your
decision-making process was hasty or unbalanced. Again, sometimes
the only way you can learn what the barriers and roadblocks are is by
running up against them. The best you can do is to learn and move forward. Apologize (Effective Apologies, page 50) if you need to (maybe
to yourself), ask for help (Clear Requests, page 48), and make a plan to
improve the situation you're in and make wiser decisions in the future.

17

reduce the impact of ADHD on your relationships

"ADHD has definitely made relationships harder, especially in my 20s. Learning to have the confidence to look for good people, relationships, and friends helps, but it took me a long time to get the courage to do that. Everyone has flaws, and knowing you're a good person is important. Get out there and find social groups that fit. Strive to keep any commitments you make to others to build trust. Disregard toxic people and work on keeping the good ones in your life. They are everywhere. And definitely learn when to keep your inner thoughts inner."

For many people, a core component of *living well* is cultivating healthy, sustaining relationships. For many people with ADHD, relationships are an important source of support and strength. At the same time, ADHD-related challenges can make it more difficult to be who you want to be in your relationships. The purpose of this chapter is to help you reflect on the ways that common ADHD-related challenges might be impacting your relationships and to direct you to some strategies—mostly in other chapters of this book.

Importantly, the purpose of this chapter is *not* to address *every possible challenge you could be facing in your relationships.* If working through this chapter leads you to the realization that you need to go deeper to address problems in your relationships, you could consider couples or family counseling (see the Resources, page 212). For marriages and intimate partnerships, I also recommend the research-backed work of Dr. John Gottman, including *The Seven Principles for Making Marriage Work* and, more recently, *Fight Right: How Successful Couples Turn Conflict into Connection,* coauthored with his wife and fellow psychologist, Dr. Julie Schwartz Gottman. For ADHD-specific resources, check out *Is It You, Me, or Adult A.D.D.?* by Gina Pera or *ADHD After Dark* by Ari Tuckman.

> **Important:** People with ADHD are more likely to find themselves in relationships that include intimate partner violence, as either the recipient or perpetrator. So **if you are feeling unsafe in any of your relationships,** reach out to the National Domestic Violence Hotline at 800-799-SAFE (7233) or text START to 88788. To repeat, this chapter is about strategies for your actions in relationships—not comprehensive help for these complex dynamics.

Self-Assessment and Roadmap

Read each statement on the facing page and choose the best answer for you by putting a checkmark (✓) in the box. Use your answers to choose which sections to review.

- *A lot* like me!—Definitely review this section!
- Somewhat like me—Review this section if you need additional ideas.
- Not like me—This section doesn't seem to apply to you, so skip it if you want.

	Not like me	Somewhat like me	*A lot* like me!	Sections to review
I don't follow through on the things I say I'm going to do, and people think I don't care.				A (page 151)
People complain that I don't listen to them.				B (page 153)
I get upset with people and say or do things I later regret.				C (page 153)
I make impulsive decisions that negatively impact people I care about.				D (page 153)
People I'm close to don't know about my ADHD or don't understand it.				E (page 153)
Someone close to me does a lot of work to help me manage my life, and I sometimes resent it or take them for granted.				F (page 155)
I'm a human being, which means no matter what, I'm going to make mistakes in my relationships.				G (page 156)

» A: I don't follow through on the things I say I'm going to do, and people think I don't care.

The following chapters might be helpful in improving follow-through with your commitments, depending on where the follow-through process breaks down for you. *Choose one* of the following that seems most relevant and start there.

If it seems right to you, tell your loved one what you're working on so that they can see and support the efforts you're making.

❑ Show Up on Time (Chapter 4)

❑ Remember and Remember to Do Things (Chapter 5)

❑ Plan and Prioritize (Chapter 7)

❑ Get Started and Restarted (Chapter 9)

❑ Stick With It and Wrap Up (Chapter 10)

❑ Keep Your Commitments to Others (Chapter 12)

In addition to these chapters, here are two strategies that might be helpful in coordinating your life with others in your family. These are two tools that my family can't function without. The first is:

❑ Shared Online Calendars

Many online calendar systems have the ability to share events. My husband, our 15-year-old, and I all keep separate Google Calendars with the ability to see the events on each other's calendars. Most helpful is the ability to invite other people to events that are relevant to them— for example, inviting my husband when I add a social event with our friends or adding my son to his scheduled dental appointments. This system prevents a lot of miscommunication and allows us to remind each other of what's coming up.

Another family organization tool is a:

❑ Household Events Calendar (page 67)

In our house, this is a small weekly whiteboard calendar posted in our kitchen. At the start of the week, we write key events from our Google calendars on the weekly whiteboard calendar, so we can all see what's coming up and identify any conflicts or overlaps. Events include social events, extracurricular activities, appointments, or any other nonroutine occurrence throughout the week. Some families use a monthly posted calendar, but we find that focusing on just the upcoming week (along with our shared Google Calendars) works well.

If you personally are struggling with follow-through, suggesting these mutual solutions to your loved ones just might benefit everyone.

≫ B: People complain that I don't listen to them.

The following Menu chapters might be helpful in this area, depending on where the process breaks down for you. Choose one that seems most relevant and start there. If it seems right to you, tell your loved ones what you're working on so that they can see and support the efforts you're making.

- ❑ Switch Gears When You Need To (manage hyperfocus) (Chapter 11)
- ❑ Absorb Information (Chapter 13)
- ❑ Make Thoughtful Decisions (Chapter 16)

≫ C: I get upset with people and say or do things I later regret.

Review the chapter below and, if it seems right to you, tell your loved ones what you're working on so that they can see and support the efforts you're making.

- ❑ Manage the Urge to Act Out When You're Upset (Chapter 15)

≫ D: I make impulsive decisions that negatively impact people I care about.

Review the chapter below and, if it seems right to you, tell your loved ones what you're working on so that they can see and support the efforts you're making.

- ❑ Make Thoughtful Decisions (Chapter 16)

≫ E: People I'm close to don't know about my ADHD or don't understand it.

Deciding to disclose your ADHD struggles is a very personal decision. It's a good idea to consider whether the person you want to talk to is equipped to respond to you in an open, supportive way. I think of it like this: Imagine you have just spent two days building a model of Notre Dame cathedral out of popsicle sticks and wood glue. (I have no idea *why* you would do this, but just go with me.) The glue has dried, so it's not too delicate, but you still have to exercise care when holding it. Would you hand your delicate creation to your 3-year-old nephew? Probably not. Likewise, you might want to be thoughtful when considering who to disclose to about your ADHD. Is this person equipped to support you? To "hold" this important information about you?

If the people in your life don't seem ready to hold your popsicle stick cathedral, there are steps you can take to open things up. Children and Adults with ADHD (CHADD) has accessible educational resources about ADHD that you can share at *https://chadd.org/for-adults/overview*. The book *When an Adult You Love Has ADHD* by Dr. Barkley might also be a resource for your family members. Skeptical folks may be more receptive if you can emphasize how your ADHD diagnosis is helping you zero in on strategies that work for you—such as the ones in this book. For example, instead of:

> *You need to understand that I don't mean to do these things—it's my ADHD.*

try:

> *I know I've had trouble keeping my word to you in the past and that's been stressful for you. I'm working on some strategies to get better at follow-through that are designed for people with ADHD. Can I tell you about what I'm working on?*

If your loved one seems receptive, you can decide whether you'd like to request some support. If you need help figuring out how to ask for it, review:

❑ Clear Requests (page 48)

Despite your best efforts, it's possible that not everyone in your life will "get" your ADHD and provide the kind of support you'd like. But for empathy and emotional support for your efforts at ADHD-related change, seek out:

❑ Support Communities (page 52)

≫ F: Someone close to me does a lot of work to help me manage my life, and I sometimes resent it or take them for granted.

This isn't necessarily a bad thing or something to be ashamed of. People bring different strengths to relationships. If your loved one's strength is executive functioning, then it's not necessarily bad if the division of labor is such that they take on more of the management tasks—so long as this arrangement is satisfying to both people and no one is feeling overtaxed or that the relationship is out of balance.

But if your answers to the questions at the beginning of this chapter led you here, you're either feeling some resentment about your loved one's level of involvement or you're worried they may be feeling overburdened. Either way, you're going to want to have a conversation with your loved one to learn more about their perspective, to share yours, and—if applicable—to renegotiate some aspects of your relationship. For example, if you feel that your loved one is overly involved in your life, you may want to ask them to check in less frequently or allow you the opportunity to try managing certain aspects of your life. If you are worried your loved one seems frustrated and overburdened, you may want to find out what they're taking on that's most stressful for them and work on some strategies to better share the load.

In planning out this conversation, it can be helpful to include the elements on page 156—a variation on the Clear Requests (page 48).

Two elements to highlight here are *expressing gratitude* and *really listening*. Expressing gratitude acknowledges the positive intent of your loved one. Really listening (Chapter 13, Section D, page 121) validates their perspective and allows you to gather information toward a solution.

Elements to Consider Including in a Conversation about Support

	Asking for less support	Offering more support
Describe the situation (just the facts).	Mom, I noticed that you call to check in on me about three times a day to make sure I'm doing what I'm supposed to.	Hon, I noticed that lately you seem more withdrawn and stressed out. I know you're doing a lot to manage everyone's schedule, including mine and the kids'.
Express gratitude.	I'm really thankful that you care so much about me and how I'm doing.	I want you to know I see this and appreciate everything that you're doing.
Give your perspective.	When you call so often, it sometimes feels like you don't trust me to handle things. Also, I can't always answer that many calls without being distracted by them.	But I feel like things are out of balance and I may not be pulling my weight here.
Ask for their perspective and *really listen* (Chapter 13, Section D, page 121).	What do you think? (Listen to understand, not respond.)	What do you think? (Listen to understand, not respond.)
Negotiate a solution.	(You may decide to have a daily check-in via text at a certain time and a weekly phone call on Sunday nights.)	(You may decide that you will take the lead on setting up a family calendar or other system to help manage scheduling load.)

» G: I'm a human being, which means no matter what, I'm going to make mistakes in my relationships.

This might just be the truest statement in this book. Even in the best relationships, people let each other down. When you are struggling with ADHD, it can be easy to feel like relationship problems are all your fault—something that you can't change. But you have the ability to take control of your part in your relationships; to seek out new, supportive people to help you be your best self; and to reduce investment in the relationships in your life that aren't serving you. And if you've hurt someone, it is never too late to apologize (Effective Apologies, page 50) and commit to positive change.

18

organize stuff and space

"I have these DOOM piles all over the place: things that I Didn't Organize, Only Moved."

People with ADHD often struggle to keep their homes, offices, desks, cars, and other physical spaces organized and neat. Home organization has become more difficult over time in the United States for most people because the average American home contains a lot more stuff than it used to. If you're reading this chapter, your struggles in this area have probably caused some problems in your life.

We're going to start this chapter a little differently for reasons that will become clear in the next section.

Examine Your Motivation

Check all the reasons below that you want to work on better organizing your spaces:

❑ My space is truly unsanitary (rotting food; pet excrement).*

❑ The disorganization means I can't find the things I need.

❑ The presence of the mess stresses me (or someone very important to me) out.

❑ I feel better when my things are organized.

❑ I'm afraid people will think less of me if they know my space
is messy.

❑ A competent person's home is neat and organized.

Why examine your reasons for wanting to be more organized?
Keeping things neat and organized will require an investment of your
time and energy, so it's good to figure out what your return on investment for these efforts is likely to be. This will help you reflect on the
extent to which your desire for organization is about *actually improving
your quality of life* compared to *meeting a perceived standard*. Reasons at the
top and middle of the list are related to quality of life, while those near
the bottom are about meeting a standard.

I will admit that I have a strong bias on this issue. My house is
almost always in some state of disorganization. I'd say it's mostly *messy*,
not dirty. We've got two kids, and they have a lot of stuff (although
it's not all their fault, to be clear), and we, overall, just have too much
stuff. On a semi-daily basis we pick up the trash, dirty dishes, and dirty
clothes and put those where they need to go. We clean obvious messes
and, from time to time, do a massive clean-out/clean-up of a particular
area. When people are coming over, we tidy and clean the spaces that
they'll see. But at this stage of our lives, that's about it.

I used to feel guilty about this. I used to think that when I eventually "got it all together" in life I'd be able to maintain a neat and tidy
house—like the aspirational *Better Homes and Gardens* magazine on our
coffee table. Growing up, I remember my mom frequently expressing
her own guilt about this issue—even though our house was far less

---

*If this describes you and you have great difficulty throwing things away and your house
is overrun with clutter, we recommend you speak with a mental health professional. You
may benefit from strategies to help people who engage in *hoarding,* an anxiety-related
disorder.

cluttered than mine is now.* But is the guilt over a messy house and the energy we use to avoid it a wise use of our resources?

My take: There is nothing morally superior about a neat and tidy house. I have decided to (mostly) stop caring unless the mess is impacting our quality of life. That's just not where we are choosing to spend our time right now, and that's okay. Of course, it is **totally valid** if you or others have different preferences about your own home. The "mess is okay" position isn't in any way superior either. Some people derive a great sense of calm and pride from having a neat home. And if you're with a partner who feels this way, you'll need to find a compromise position and respect their preferences too. But *it's up to you to decide what matters.*

Set Your Priorities

Examining your motivations to get organized can help you set your priorities. Which physical spaces will you spend your time and energy on? You're more likely to be successful if you focus on making specific changes in one area. Maybe it's your messy bedroom that stresses you out or a disorganized desk that's causing you to waste time looking for things. To figure this out, gather some data by doing an:

❑ Organization Audit

Take a day or two and, as you move through the spaces in your life, take note of where disorganized spaces cause problems for you. Then answer the following questions:

Which disorganized spaces in your life cause you the most problems? Consider the time you take searching for things and any conflicts that the mess causes in your life.

---

* In most families, the burden of housework and the stigma of a messy house falls disproportionately on women.

_____

_____

_____

_____

Looking back at your list, which space do you want to focus on first? You can choose based on what's causing the most problems or where you feel like change is the most possible.

I'll focus on: _____

_____

Next, based on your observations, identify **three changes** in this space that would improve things the most. Here's an example for my bedroom:

- Keep clothes and shoes off the floor—in hamper, hung up/on shoe rack, or on the "transition chair"*
- Keep dresser drawers closed (reason: open drawers specifically annoy my usually chill husband)
- Keep jewelry items off dresser top

Below, write down your three changes for the space you identified:

1. _____

2. _____

3. _____

---

*This is a chair where I put clothing items that could be worn again before washing. I used to feel guilty about this chair until I heard an organization expert on a podcast praise it as a practice that helps the environment!

Engineer Your Environment

The way you set up your spaces will influence whether you will maintain your changes. A key idea here is to place objects in your physical space at the *point of performance*. Put more simply, you'll set up your spaces so that you have what you need when and where you want an action to happen. This is a variation on the idea of a prompt (page 23) For example, if you always get undressed in your bathroom, put your dirty clothes hamper . . . in the bathroom, not in a completely separate room. If you need a spatula 90% of the time you cook on your stove, put the spatulas in a crock by the stove, not in a drawer on the other side of the kitchen. An example I shared earlier in the book from a former student is putting your condiments in the refrigerator crisper drawers and your fresh produce on the door shelves, so you'll see it and use it more easily. Little "nudges" like this can increase the efficiency of your behavior and reduce the load on your self-regulation.

I take inspiration from pioneering industrial psychologist Lillian Gilbreth, who designed the modern kitchen by observing how real users interacted with their environment. Gilbreth *invented* those refrigerator door shelves as well as the step trash can and the standard kitchen counter height. I encourage you to be your own Lillian Gilbreth and get excited about the ways you could set up your environment to make your life more efficient.

In engineering your environment, another useful idea is the *desire path*. In the field of design and engineering, a desire path is some indication in the environment of how people are naturally using the space. For example, people may cut across a lawn from one sidewalk to the other, literally wearing a path through the grass. Designers observe this and then may modify the walkway to fit the desire path. You can be on the lookout for desire paths in your home as well. *Where* do you drop your clothes when they don't make it to the hamper? Put the hamper there. On what flat surface are you leaving stray items? Put a tray or bin there. Observing desire paths won't solve all your problems, but it will make sticking with changes easier. Also, I find it pretty fun.

Here are a few ideas to consider as you engineer your environment:

- Create Home Bases (see Chapter 6, page 72) for items you lose a lot and put the Home Base in a location where it's easy to use—for example, a hook for your keys right inside the door.

- Put a bin or tray on flat surfaces where you often leave things.

- Put needed items where you can most easily grab them—for example, empty hangers all together at the end of the rack.

- Put a car-sized trash can in the spot in your car where you find empty food wrappers.

For your three target changes, consider the idea of *point of performance* and *desire paths* and make any changes to your environment to support the behavior you want to see. Write your engineering moves here:

_____

_____

_____

Get Rid of Stuff

The less stuff you have, the less stuff you have to manage. This topic could be—and is!—the subject of entire books. Recently, some adults with ADHD on TikTok have recommended taking each object and asking themselves, if it were covered with poop, would you clean it and keep it? If not, get rid of it. This tactic of associating disgust with an item can force you to decide whether you really want to keep something.

If the thought of sorting through all your DOOM piles seems overwhelming, don't just toss out the entire pile of stuff (known as "tossing"), as some people on Dr. Barkley's YouTube channel said they did with much regret. There are often important items in there (like a passport, phone charger, cash or credit cards, and so on). So start with the Rule of 10 or the Two-Minute Rule: Set the goal of acting on 10 separate items—keep/donate/throw away—or set a timer for 2 minutes and do the same. Then move on to doing something else for a bit, coming back to do another chunk later. (Timers will be *very* helpful here.) Being an indiscriminate "tosser," getting so fed up with your DOOM piles that you throw all the stuff out, could lead to your inadvertently tossing important things you need.

I also recommend this concise, humorous, and helpful article in *The New Yorker* by Patricia Marx: *www.newyorker.com/magazine/2022/02/28/a-guide-to-getting-rid-of-almost-everything-decluttering.* Among Marx's recommendations, I'd like to highlight the amazingness of *gifting economies*. These are groups set up on online platforms like Facebook where people freely gift unwanted items to others, request free items, and express gratitude for the gifts they receive. You can always sell your stuff on Craigslist or Facebook Marketplace or take a load of stuff to your local charity thrift store (and please do), but there can be something uniquely rewarding and satisfying about knowing you are generously fulfilling someone's specific need by getting rid of your stuff. I am a member of a hyperlocal Facebook group like this—a *gifting group*—and I have been able to get rid of lots of unwanted items and pick up some things I actually need.* (And if I don't end up needing them, I pass them back to the group.) Freecycle is another popular online platform for gifting. No matter what method you choose, do some stuff purging and you will have less to manage.

Build the Habit: Tidying Rituals

Returning to the three changes you identified on page 161, the last step—and frankly the most difficult—is to start building the habitual behavior that will maintain the change. What's going to remind you to keep up with your changes? It helps to think of establishing *tidying rituals* to maintain organization. If you can tag your tidying to

---

*This group started out as a Buy Nothing group, but Buy Nothing has changed a lot and is now an app instead of a local gifting movement. Try searching Facebook for "gifting group" as that's what many of these groups changed their names to.

certain times of day or certain other events in your life, it will help you remember to tidy and move this behavior from having to think about it consciously to an automatic habit. In particular, you can use Alarms, Reminders, and Prompts (page 23) to help cue the behavior.

For example, here are tidying rituals I could develop for my three target changes, along with a reminder:

- Keep clothes and shoes off the floor—put these items in the hamper, on the rack, or on the "transition chair" right away. Just before bed, scan the floor and put stray on-the-floor items where they go.
- Keep dresser drawers closed—do this whenever you walk away from the dresser and during your before-bed check.
- Keep jewelry items off your dresser top—put items directly in the tray during before-bed check.
- Post a reminder on your bedroom or bathroom mirror of the three things that should happen during before-bed check.

Write out your tidying rituals for each of the three changes you identified. Be sure to consider how you could use Alarms, Reminders, and Prompts to cue the behavior.

_____

_____

_____

When You Just Need to *Blitz Clean*

Sometimes you just need to do what I call *blitz cleaning* and give a space a full overhaul—like before a party or when you (or your partner) just can't stand the clutter another moment. But sometimes you just feel *so tired*. You need some strategies to get moving. In these cases, any of the strategies in Chapter 9 could be applied to cleaning and organizing:

❏ Get Started and Restarted

For example, you could set a timer for 10 minutes and see how much you and your other family members can tidy in that time. Another thing our family does is employ one of those currently popular three-level rolling craft carts. Someone is tasked with walking around the house picking up stray items and putting them in the cart. When the cart is full, the person goes through the items and either throws them out or puts them back where they belong. And instead of one big "junk drawer," we have an old library card catalog, and we put small items in each labeled drawer—such as pens, paper clips, batteries, rulers, and so on. It's kind of fun to sort the items, and we always know where we can find these things without digging through a drawer. I share these examples because they illustrate the creative solutions that are possible to help manage your stuff. Get excited about what you might discover!

19

find your fit at work or school

"After working in restaurant jobs for 20-plus years, I finally found my career path—it was working with dogs. First, I was a dog walker. Then I became a dog trainer and behavior consultant. This has been such a great fit for me. I also found that I love giving group lessons to dog owners, which was a huge surprise because I don't like public speaking. I find leading these groups so much fun: It's active, the people come and go, so I get to meet new people and dogs and work with them—so there is continuing novelty. I also get to (over)share what I know, and I am providing much needed support to the owners and their dogs. Networking with lots of other dog-related professionals has led me to believe that many people who have chosen this career are probably neurodivergent."

Most people in industrialized nations spend the majority of their lives learning in school and working at a formal job. ADHD can have a profound impact on both of these areas of life, so this chapter is designed to zero in on problems in these areas. However, keep in mind that the entire rest of this book contains skills that could help with specific problems at work or school. Here we will focus on some issues not covered elsewhere.

Self-Assessment and Roadmap

Read each statement below and choose the best answer for you by putting a checkmark (✓) in the box. Use your answers to choose which sections to review.

- *A lot* like me!—Definitely review this section!
- Somewhat like me—Review this section if you need additional ideas.
- Not like me—This section doesn't seem to apply to you, so skip it if you want.

	Not like me	Somewhat like me	*A lot* like me!	Sections to review
I think my job or what I'm studying in school might not be the best fit for my strengths and weaknesses—including my ADHD-related challenges.				A (page 168)
I think some modifications to my work or school environment could help me function better.				B (page 172)
I'm afraid ADHD is going to prevent me from having the degree or career I really want.				C (page 175)

>> A: I think my job or what I'm studying in school might not be the best fit for my strengths and weaknesses—including my ADHD-related challenges.

Congratulations on having the wisdom to step back and reflect on whether your current path is the right one! Seriously, this is hard to do because it seems like everyone (at least in the United States) is expected to have a quick and confident answer to the question "What do you do?" or "What are you studying in school?" When you're young, you can feel a lot of pressure to get on a well-defined track and follow it—whether that's the track you really want, the track that your parents expect of you, or the track that's simply most convenient to get on at the moment. Switching gears can be difficult—but *if done thoughtfully, with self-awareness and a good plan,* it can offer benefits. Especially if you get on a path that's a better fit for your strengths and values.

Finding a good fit at work and school may be even more important for people with ADHD. The self-regulation challenges that accompany the disorder make it difficult for some people to do well in "traditional" work environments—like "desk jobs" that require intense focus or less structured environments that require a lot of self-direction. One adult with ADHD pointed out something that I think is very valuable: that it's really important to find a job that aligns with your values and ethics. Paying attention and controlling your impulses is even harder when you're doing something that requires you to go against your moral compass.

In psychology, finding your fit is known as *niche picking,* which is when people seek out environments that work best with their characteristics. So you can think of the process of identifying better-fitting careers as *finding your niche.* Not everyone would be an equally good fit for every job or program, so just because you've run into problems in your current career doesn't mean there might not be a better niche out there for you. The challenge of course is to figure out what niches might be a better fit and how to get into them.

❑ Begin to Reflect.

Start by reflecting on the following:

What are some things that you really care about? What gives you a sense of accomplishment?

_____

_____

_____

What are some things that you could do for hours without
outside prompting?

_____

_____

_____

_____

What are you are good at? What are your strengths (so far)?

_____

_____

_____

_____

Have you had any work or volunteer experiences that you
really enjoyed or felt successful at? What was it about them that
appealed to you?

_____

_____

_____

_____

Where and when do you like to work? Do you prefer to be
outdoors or indoors? Physically moving or sitting? Interacting
with people or solitary? A 9-to-5 or a changing work schedule?
Traveling or staying put?

_____

_____

_____

_____

Did you notice anything interesting or surprising about what you wrote? Of course, *not everything you find enjoyable that you're good at is a viable pathway to supporting yourself financially.*★ But identifying *elements* of a career that might appeal to your strengths can point you in some useful directions you might not have thought of otherwise.

❑ Take it to the pros.

Finding your niche may be a lifelong journey, but there are people who are trained to help you along the way. Next, you might set up an appointment with a professional career counselor. Take along your answers to the questions above and begin the process. Why? Professionals are aware of more career fields than you can even imagine, and they know which of these fields are in demand and what the training requirements are.

If you're in the United States, you can get **free career counseling** through American Job Centers. These government-funded centers provide a range of job services under one roof, including career counseling. Visit *www.careeronestop.org/LocalHelp/AmericanJobCenters/ find-american-job-centers.aspx* to find a center near you. (I found four centers within a 25-mile radius of my house.) Also, if you are an alumnus of a college or university, you may be able to receive career services through your university's career center. Something to check out! And for ideas as well as inspiration, Google "ADHD success stories" to see the myriad celebrities, athletes, musicians, entrepreneurs, and others who have done very well despite having ADHD.

When you have identified some fields of interest, next **talk to people who actually do that work.** Unless you've done a job, you probably don't see all the day-to-day details and, potentially, the not-so-fun aspects of that career. (Ask me about being a professor and how we supposedly "get the summers off.") They can also give you the best advice about how to pursue their line of work. How can you find someone to talk to? The career center could help, but the easiest way

---

★ At one point in college, I nearly followed the path to being a professional classical singer. Because of the degree of "hustle" needed to be a professional musician and the uncertainty of securing your next gig, I decided I wanted it to be my lifelong amateur passion, and that was the right choice for me.

might be to search for message boards related to that field on sites like Reddit and post some questions about that career area.* You can also "cold email" people in that field who have their contact information posted online (email me about being a professor!) or ask around in your social network.

Once you have identified the niche you'd like to pick, you'll probably need to use the tools in other parts of this book to set goals, make a plan, and take the next step. The following chapters may be particularly helpful:

❑ Plan and Prioritize (Chapter 7)

❑ Get Started and Restarted (Chapter 9)

❑ Stick with It and Wrap Up (Chapter 10)

❑ Make Thoughtful Decisions (Chapter 16)

≫ B: I think some modifications to my work or school environment could help me function better.

In the United States, adults with ADHD may qualify for *reasonable accommodations* in higher education or the workplace under the Americans with Disabilities Act (ADA). An accommodation is an adjustment to the environment or to a task—for example, installing a wheelchair ramp, providing reading materials in Braille, or allowing work to be performed in a quiet office space. In higher education, a common accommodation is allowing additional time to complete a test if a person's disability affects their mental processing speed. In educational settings the purpose of an accommodation is to allow a person with a disability to have equal access to and participation in a school's programs. In the workplace, accommodations allow a person with a disability who is otherwise qualified for the job to perform its essential functions.

Because the ADA is a federal law, there's a lot of nitty-gritty when it comes to the terminology and details about who qualifies and what

---

*Don't just read posts from people in the field, because they may just be venting. Be sure to ask a question that allows people to talk about both the pros and the cons.

institutions are required to do. I recommend this web page by CHADD, which does a nice job of parsing the legalese: *https://chadd.org/for-adults/legal-rights-in-higher-education-and-the-workplace*. In addition, ADA information specialists are ready to answer your questions via a confidential national toll-free hotline at 1-800-949-4232 (Monday–Friday, 9:00 A.M.–5:00 P.M., Eastern).

Before deciding to request accommodations:

- Think about what aspects of ADHD interfere most with your ability to access your education or perform your job duties.
- Then think about what adjustments to your environment or tasks could help. Some of the ideas you encounter in other parts of this book might be great accommodations!
- If you do identify solutions, you may be able to ask to put these in place without formally requesting accommodations. However, if you need adjustments that involve major changes to the physical environment or exceptions to class or company policy, you will likely need to make a formal request.

Accommodations in Higher Education

In higher education, accommodations are intended to allow a person with disabilities to have equal access to their educational program. Accommodations don't involve changes to academic standards or program requirements. For example, students might receive an accommodation of taking their test in a place with fewer distractions than the classroom, but they would take exactly the same test. This web page from the Department of Education describes the process for requesting accommodations: *www2.ed.gov/about/offices/list/ocr/transition.html*. Here's a step-by-step outline:

1. **Find out what your school requires to request accommodations.** Most schools have a disability services office or coordinator, and information about the process should be available on their website. If not, a quick email should point you in the right direction. For example, here is the web page for the University of Richmond's

Disability Services Office: *https://disability.richmond.edu*. Review the available information about your school's requirements to receive accommodations and take notes.

2. **Get your documentation.** Schools vary in the documentation they will require to verify your need for accommodations. Many schools will require you to provide a psychological evaluation report or doctor's letter that verifies that you have a disability and makes the case for specific accommodations. This step can be lengthy and, if you haven't received a formal evaluation and your school requires it, costly as well. Other schools may accept less formal documentation or, for example, an Individualized Education Program (IEP) from high school.

3. **Request your accommodations.** The school will have a process for submitting your documentation and making your request. Some schools will have you meet with a counselor in their office to discuss which accommodations might be most helpful; for others you'll need to do your homework to determine what might be best.

4. **Discuss accommodations with professors.** At most schools, each semester you will be provided with documentation of your accommodations that you can give to each of your professors. This documentation will *not* say that you have ADHD; rather, it will outline the accommodations you have been granted. Because each course has its own structure and policies, it's good to have a meeting with each professor to discuss how best to arrange the accommodation in their class. For example, if a class has 10-minute quizzes at the start of each class period and you have been granted "time and a half" testing time, you may need to get to class 5 minutes early to start your quizzes.

5. **Troubleshoot as needed.** If you have any difficulty getting your approved accommodations, circle back to your disability services office or coordinator, who can help negotiate solutions.

Accommodations in the Workplace

Requesting and obtaining workplace accommodations for ADHD is an area that I will admit I am much less familiar with. I also think the process is less standardized than it is for higher education settings, which tend to have administrative offices devoted to managing such requests. If your workplace has a human resources department, this is where you would go to get the accommodations process started. If not, the process is likely to be less formalized. As in higher education, requesting accommodations in the workplace will likely require that you obtain documentation of your disability and need for accommodations from a health care provider, which may require a formal evaluation if you have not already had one.

But beware: It is wise to "assess the room" by determining how disability friendly and accommodating your workplace has been to others before disclosing your own ADHD. There are numerous stories on Dr. Barkley's YouTube channel on this topic (Should You Disclose Your ADHD to Your Employer?) of people disclosing ADHD to their employers only to be targeted for various complaints and eventually fired or otherwise treated poorly by their supervisors. Moreover, the adults sharing their stories remind others that the HR department works for the employer and is not always your best friend or therapist. While they may be there to provide some help to you, they also exist to protect the employer from legal infringements or violations and from accusations of workplace discrimination. So think before you leap into disclosing and asking for work accommodations.

For further information and guidance, visit the wonderfully comprehensive website by the Equal Employment Opportunity Commission (EEOC)—the Job Accommodation Network at *https://askjan.org*. The "For Individuals" section offers comprehensive information about how to request accommodations. In addition, there's a wealth of information on possible accommodations for ADHD and other disabilities in their searchable database: *https://askjan.org/a-to-z.cfm*. Accommodation ideas there include Reduced-Distraction Environments, more frequent check-ins, and assigning a mentor.

>> **C: I'm afraid ADHD is going to prevent me from having the degree or career I really want.**

This is a really, really hard feeling to carry. If you didn't care deeply about this direction in your life, it wouldn't cause you pain to think about not reaching this goal. I don't have *answers* here—just thoughts to share.

Begin by recognizing that this fear is the *story that you're telling yourself.* (See also Section D in Chapter 15.) That story may be based on solid evidence from your past experience, but your life is still being lived, and so there is always the possibility of meeting your goals. You don't have to let your past become your future.* By reading this book, you're already making an investment in what you *can* control about that future to move toward your goals.

Taking a closer look at the story you are writing for yourself, I invite you consider what you've identified as the *successful ending* to this story. Perhaps your *successful ending* is earning a PhD in history, becoming a veterinarian, or owning your own successful restaurant. These are goals that only a small percentage of people achieve in their lifetimes. Let me be clear: There is *nothing wrong* with setting high goals for what you want in your life. But even if your goals are modest compared to other people's, I would like to gently suggest that one way of living well is to cultivate the idea of *many successful endings* throughout the course of your life story.

I am about to get personal here. I never expected—in fact, I had feared—becoming the mom of a child with special needs on the autism spectrum. Yet parenting my son has revealed to me the bullshit I had believed about what counts as a *successful ending* for my story and, most importantly, for his. I also realized how narrowly I had previously defined what counted as success for a person.** Among many other gifts, my kiddo has given me the gift of more flexible thinking about what a person really needs to live a life of value.

Figuring out what values underlie your goals is the key to defining *many successful endings.*

---

*I keep a sign on my desk at work that helps me when I get in this mode that reads, "Don't stumble over something behind you."

**If you want, you can see a lecture I gave that includes some of these ideas (*https://youtu. be/Oky59qjjuys*). It's called a "Last Lecture," where you're asked to give the lecture you'd give if you knew it was your last. Heavy stuff!

What is the degree or career you really want—the one that led you to this section? Write it here and be specific:

_____

_____

_____

_____

What specifically is it about this degree or career pathway that makes you want to pursue it? What's your *why?*

_____

_____

_____

_____

Look back at your answers and reflect: What does the fact that you have this educational or career goal tell you about what you value? Here are some examples to illustrate:

- Earning a PhD in history might represent a commitment to deep learning, to helping people understand the relevance of the past to the future, or to contributing new knowledge to the world.

- Becoming a veterinarian might represent a commitment to the well-being of animals and the natural world, to being there for other people in their times of need, or to challenging yourself to continuously learn new skills.

- Owning your own successful restaurant might represent a commitment to bringing joy to people through food, fostering culinary creativity, or being an important part of your local community.

Your turn: What might your goal be telling you about what you value?

_____

_____

_____

Finally, begin to imagine what *other successful endings* could be. In other words, what other degrees or career directions could move you toward the values you identified? For example, the aspiring history PhD might also find value in work as an educator at a historical site. The aspiring vet might also find value in work as an animal behavior specialist helping to rehome pets who have experienced abuse. The aspiring restaurateur might also find value in working for a community-lending nonprofit that helps small restaurant owners secure capital.

What are your ideas for other successful endings?

_____

_____

_____

What did you notice? You might notice that you identify some things you could actually get involved in *right now* to move in the direction of your values! (Which is pretty cool. It's not just about the ending—if we think creatively, there's a way to live in our values every day, at every moment.) Exercises like this can also help you decide what opportunities to say yes to and which ones to let pass.

What next? As you pursue the *successful ending* of your heart's desire, I encourage you to remain flexible and open to what other successful endings might look like for you.

If you found the work in this chapter valuable (see what I did there?), you might consider exploring Chapter 26 (What Are Your *Why*s?) and Chapter 27 (The Principles) in Part Three.

= 20 =

eat well

"My biggest problems are in knowing what to do and not doing it, but also it's more in the timing and pacing of eating. It's very easy for me to go through an entire day going from one task to another, saying 'I'll eat lunch after I do this one thing,' and then bam—it'll be evening, and I haven't had a glass of water or scrap of food all day. I'm then ravenous in the evening, which is the worst time of day to metabolize even good food."

While there's no evidence that certain diets are the cause of or cure for ADHD, there is ample evidence that it's considerably harder for adults with ADHD to practice good nutrition due to problems with impulsivity and self-regulation. When it comes to specific recommendations, there is some evidence that omega-3 fatty acids found in foods such as salmon might have some limited benefits for some people with ADHD. And if taken in the recommended doses, they are unlikely to cause harm, so these might be something to consider. While there are countless diets and eating styles that people swear by, some common themes of a healthy diet include limiting processed foods high in fat and sugar and making sure to consume foods with sufficient vitamins, minerals, protein, and fiber. I recommend that you consult your physician or a nutritionist regarding what's best for your dietary needs.

Eating better is a tough topic for a lot of people for a lot of good reasons. First, for a lot of people, there's a lot of guilt and shame tied up with our decisions about what we eat. Second, eating healthy is very hard because healthier food is expensive while less healthy food is often cheaper, easy to get, requires little preparation, and is engineered by corporations to taste good. So if you have any guilt about food choices, it's time to let it go because one reason you may struggle is that the environment is set up to work against you.

But fortunately, you can also modify your environment in ways that will set you up for eating well.

If you want to make some changes in your eating practices, it can be a good idea to consult with a nutritionist to get more information about good choices for you and to set some goals.

One strategy they might recommend for learning more about your eating is to keep a food log. You can do this by writing down what you eat using pencil and paper, but I recommend using one of the many apps available for food tracking, such as Calorie King or My Fitness Pal. When I track my food, it's always eye-opening and informative, increasing my awareness of what I'm actually eating and then forgetting about.

Consider framing your eating goals positively, as in what you will eat **more** of instead of just what you should eat less of. What nutritious foods do you already like to eat or ones you'd like to try?

Once you set your eating goals in consultation with a professional, the tools described in the prior chapters may be helpful toward reaching your goals.

Ask yourself:

*When I **don't** eat in line with my health goals, where am I getting off track?*

Based on your answer, choose a chapter to review that might provide some useful tips and insights.

❑ Remember and Remember to Do Things (Chapter 5)
❑ Plan and Prioritize (Chapter 7)

❑ Get Started and Restarted (Chapter 9)

❑ Make Thoughtful Decisions (Chapter 16)

These Toolbox items might also be helpful for moments when your eating doesn't line up with your goals:

❑ Alarms, Reminders, and Prompts (page 23)

❑ Accountability Partners (page 33)

❑ Choice Point Analysis (page 36)

❑ Self-Coaching (page 40)

❑ Moments of Mindfulness (page 44)

❑ Emotional Antidotes (page 46)

❑ Speed Bumps (page 47)

A Note about Dietary Supplements

Is it just me, or are ads for dietary supplements everywhere lately? It seems as though every celebrity or influencer is selling their own formulation of "natural" supplements to help with mood, focus, digestion, sleep, and so on. While supplements often seem like a side-effect-free option or a safer alternative to prescription drugs, because they're not studied and regulated like drugs, there's good reason to be cautious when deciding whether to use them.

Consider the following:

- Dietary supplement companies don't have to show that their products work. Unlike drugs, the Food and Drug Administration (FDA) doesn't require supplement companies to submit any evidence of effectiveness.

- Dietary supplement companies don't have to show that their products are safe. Unlike drugs, the FDA doesn't require supplement companies to submit evidence of safety. Rather, safety concerns might get reported only after the supplements hit the market.

- Dietary supplements, like any substance, can and do have side effects—especially when taken in higher doses than the body has evolved to handle.

- Dietary supplements often don't contain what's advertised. Studies have shown that supplements often don't contain the doses of ingredients advertised on the label and, in some cases, don't include listed ingredients at all.

- Dietary supplements can have problematic interactions with each other and with medications. *It's important to tell your doctor if you're taking any dietary supplements.*

There are ways to be a savvy consumer of dietary supplements. Visit *www.quality-supplements.org*, a website by the nonprofit U.S. Pharmacopeial Convention, an industry group that lists dietary supplements that have met standards higher than those required by the FDA. Most of all, ask yourself: Why am I taking this supplement? What do I know about whether these ingredients actually help the problem I'm taking them for? Then chat with your doctor.

21

sleep well

"When you're interested in everything, sleep can feel like a punishment!"

You probably know firsthand how groggy and foggy you get when you haven't had sufficient sleep—that hollow-eyed, brittle feeling after pulling an all-nighter. But even milder forms of sleep deprivation, such as chronically being short of the hours you need or ongoing poor-quality sleep, can reduce your ability to pay attention and regulate your emotions.

Here are three evidence-based recommendations to consider:

1. **Keep bedtimes and wake times as consistent as possible** regardless of day of the week. Sleep researchers have started to use the term *social jet lag* to describe the negative effects of a sleep schedule that bounces all around the clock.

2. **Control your bedtime exposure to screens.** I know first-hand how using a phone or tablet in bed can lead to endless, mindless scrolling that delays sleep and interferes with circadian rhythm. See Switch Gears When You Need To (Chapter 11), Section C, for specific ideas on how to manage this.

3. **Talk to your doctor** if your sleep problems persist. A sleep study might be a good option for you. This type of assessment

sometimes reveals underlying factors, such as sleep apnea, that may severely reduce the positive effects of sleep and even cause symptoms that mimic ADHD.

   If you want even more evidence-based recommendations for working on your sleep, the U.K. National Health Service has published a **free online self-help program** based on cognitive-behavioral therapy that can educate you about sleep and help you start making changes: *www.nhsinform.scot/illnesses-and-conditions/mental-health/mental-health-self-help-guides/sleep-problems-and-insomnia-self-help-guide.*

22

watch your substance use

"In the past, I think my substance use was a coping mechanism for my ADHD symptoms to some degree—but one that ended up causing more problems in the long run. I didn't necessarily realize that at the time."

Throughout most of history, humans have been using nonfood substances to alter their brain functioning. Modern prescription drugs for focusing attention or boosting mood are a very recent extension of these practices. If you're like many adults with ADHD, you might use alcohol, nicotine, or marijuana regularly—maybe even daily. I'm not here to preach to you about substance use, but to encourage you to consider whether your current use could be excessive, as it can be for many adults with ADHD, and having any negative impacts on your ADHD symptoms or your health in general. Despite claims to the contrary, all these substances can have negative effects under certain conditions.

At the same time, most of these substances aren't inherently good or bad—it all depends on how often you're using them, how much, how you're getting them into your body, and why you're using. For example, if you're using alcohol every night to help you sleep, it might be time to ask your doctor about a sleep study or other assessment to get to the bottom of your sleep issues. If you're using marijuana daily to manage stress and anxiety, it could be time to get a psychological assessment to identify anxiety treatment options. If you're vaping all day to stay focused, maybe it's time to talk to your doctor about your ADHD medication dose.

The bottom line is that it's never a bad thing to reflect honestly on your substance use and get more information about what your use might be telling you about your needs. When it comes to your ADHD medication, you should always take it at the prescribed dose, at the prescribed time, and put it into your body in the prescribed way—for the most part, swallowing a pill. If you are experiencing problems misusing ADHD medication or any other substance, help is available. If you or someone you know is concerned about your use of substances, talk to your doctor or, if in the United States, you can call the Substance Abuse and Mental Health Services Administrations (SAMHSA) National Helpline at 1-800-662-HELP(4357). The service is a confidential, free, 24-hour-a-day, 365-day-a-year information service, in English and Spanish, for individuals and family members facing mental and/or substance use disorders. You can also text your 5-digit ZIP code to 435748 (HELP4U) to receive free referral information.

23

move your body

"Exercise without a doubt gives me a very noticeable reduction in ADHD symptoms. I've seen similar results with both cardio, like running or swimming, and weight lifting. The benefits seem to last for one or two days after the exercise."

Ah! Everyone's favorite subject: exercise. If you already have a regular exercise practice, it's likely that you already know the ways it benefits you, including positive effects on your ADHD symptoms. Some people with ADHD report that regular, vigorous exercise is absolutely essential to managing their ADHD. And regardless of the impacts of exercise on ADHD, the general health benefits of moving your body regularly are undeniable.

Sometimes people wonder what the best kind of exercise is for ADHD. At this point, the answer is "we don't really know." There are a few studies showing that high-intensity interval training—engaging in very vigorous activity in short bursts—may be particularly helpful for people with ADHD, but the evidence is still pretty slim. Of course, you should consult your doctor before beginning any exercise program.

I strongly believe that *the best exercise is the exercise that you don't hate to do.* I cannot emphasize this enough. If you hate to run, you should not try to "make yourself" do it because somehow it feels more legitimate than other kinds of exercise. Sure, there are people who learn to love running, but my guess is that the number of those people who exist is vastly outstripped by the number of people who gave it up and felt bad about it. There is no shame in disliking a particular form of exercise. When it comes to exercise, you've got to set yourself up for success.

Anything that gets your body moving for an extended period of time is a good place to start. Expand your idea of what "working out" could be. I basically didn't exercise regularly until I stumbled into a dance fitness program (Jazzercise) and got hooked on the moves, the music, and the community. I know of a woman who had never exercised regularly but took up crew (rowing) in her 50s, joined a team, and got hooked. One key element in both these examples is that the exercise occurred alongside or in collaboration with other people, so you might want to consider whether working out with others would be something you would enjoy and might increase your accountability. Regardless, get creative and open-minded about what you might try.

Even if you come to enjoy your workouts, it can be incredibly difficult to carve out the time to engage regularly. Use the prompts below to get started:

> What kind of exercise or workout do you want to try? If it requires attending a class, program, or facility, look up some information about where and when you can do it.
>
> _____
>
> _____
>
> When will you do this exercise in the next week? Put it in your calendar with a reminder and the location of the facility (if applicable).
>
> _____
>
> _____

Finally, go through Get Started and Restarted (Chapter 9) with an eye toward identifying tools that could help you stick to your exercise goals. I believe in you!

24

manage money

> "My financial life used to be a catastrophe—even though I have a degree in finance! Before, I was always in debt, no matter how much I earned. I had to face up to the reality that my issue wasn't not having enough money; it was my habits that needed changing."

Managing money over the long haul is one big self-regulation exercise, which is why so many people struggle in this area of their lives. Buying a latte today versus saving and investing that five bucks might not seem like a big deal, but small daily choices add up. If you need help in this area, here's what I recommend.

1. Get Educated

An essential first step in managing your money better is to educate yourself about personal finance—something that, frustratingly, isn't taught well in schools. Start by choosing one of the two free online courses described below.* Even if you don't end up completing the

---

*Special thanks to my son Liam for his assistance in reviewing these courses.

entire course, covering some of the basic modules will give you a foundation to move forward.

- **Financial Planning for Young Adults:** *www.coursera.org/learn/financial-planning*. This eight-module highly rated online course by the University of Illinois on the Coursera platform offers an introduction to personal finance for beginners or a refresher for anyone. (Not just useful for young adults!) Completing the entire course takes about 20 hours at your own pace, and it includes high-quality and engaging video lectures, interactive discussion boards, and other resources related to each topic. You can get access to these materials for free by auditing the course. However, if you want access to quizzes and assignments and to receive a certificate of completion, the cost is about $50. Auditing this course would be great for people who really enjoy learning through videos and who mostly want information about the topics rather than practice exercises.

- **Financial Literacy by Khan Academy:** *www.khanacademy.org/college-careers-more/financial-literacy*. This 14-unit course by the well-regarded Khan Academy program includes shorter videos interspersed with articles, interactive activities, and short quizzes to check your understanding. Each module ends with a unit test to confirm your retention of the material. Completing this course will take a little longer than the Coursera course, as it is a bit more comprehensive in breadth of topics. However, the Coursera course tends to go a little more in depth on each topic. This course would be best for learners who like a lot of interaction with the platform to stay engaged and who want to boost their memory for what they have learned.

2. Track Your Spending

To know where your financial problem areas are, you're going to need to figure out where exactly your money is going. Technology has made money easier to spend, but it has also made that spending easier to track. Here are some ideas for figuring out what you're spending, where.

- **Information online from your bank.** Your bank might already provide you with helpful online tools to track your spending; however, if you spend from sources not linked to your bank, you might be missing crucial information.

- **Spending tracking and budgeting apps.** Link your accounts to these apps, which can track your spending and sort it into categories as well as offer tools for budgeting, saving, and other tasks. Two apps getting positive reviews are:

  o PocketGuard, recently rated by the *Wall Street Journal* as the best money tracking and budgeting app for beginners.* You can get a free trial for a week, after which the cost is $75 per year if you pay all at once or $156 if you pay month to month.

  o Rocket Money recently topped CNET's list of money management apps.** It offers a basic account for free (although reviews say it's pretty bare bones). The Premium version has a free week trial and then costs $48 a year if paying all at once and $144 a year if paying month to month. I signed up and immediately found a $12.99 per month subscription I had forgotten about and wasn't using, so for me the app paid for itself immediately!

- **Spreadsheets!** If you don't want to spend money on . . . something to help you track your money, there are lots of free spreadsheet templates online that can help you get started: *www.tillerhq.com/free-google-sheets-budget-templates*. You'll need to go on the hunt for all your statements to fill in the blanks.

3. Make a Budget

Use the resources available in the app you chose or the budgeting steps you learned about in step 1 above (Get Educated) to set your budget goals.

---

* *www.wsj.com/buyside/personal-finance/financial-tips/best-budgeting-apps*

** *www.cnet.com/personal-finance/banking/advice/best-budgeting-apps*

4. Apply Skills to Problem-Spending Areas

Now, using your budget, identify your biggest problem area of spending. Are you:

- Making big, impulsive purchases you can't afford?
- Hanging on to a big, recurring expense—like high rent or an expensive car payment?
- Making small, daily purchases—like a morning latte—that are hard to resist and don't seem like a big deal . . . until they add up?
- Spending on eating out and food delivery that's draining your bank account, and you need to learn how to cook at home more often?

Look at your spending and ask this question:

When I'm not saving and spending in line with my goals, what's going wrong?

_____

_____

Based on what you've discovered about your problem areas, choose a Toolbox tool or Menu chapter to apply to this area:

- ❑ Alarms, Reminders, and Prompts (page 23)
- ❑ Accountability Partners (page 33)
- ❑ Choice Point Analysis (page 36)
- ❑ Self-Coaching (page 40)
- ❑ Speed Bumps (page 47)
- ❑ Support Communities (page 52)
- ❑ Switch Gears When You Need To (Chapter 11)
- ❑ Make Thoughtful Decisions (Chapter 16)

25

drive safely

"The past few years (I'm 35) I've had to be very deliberate in managing distractions while I am driving. I have been fortunate not to have been arrested, but I have had serious crashes. I have developed some self-control by getting distractions out of my car and by knowing my triggers for speeding and even road rage (emotions and fatigue)."

Because people with ADHD struggle with distractibility and impulsivity, it's not surprising that they have more problems driving safely than the average adult. If safe driving has been a struggle for you, consider the following strategies:

• **Take your prescribed meds before driving** (see the Resources, page 212). Medications work "from the outside in" to reduce your symptoms and, as a result, your risk of car accidents.

• **Block access to cell phone use.** Distracted driving is one of the leading causes of accidents, regardless of whether you have ADHD. Put your phone in the back seat while driving or use tech solutions that limit phone functions while driving, such as AT&T's DriveMode app or *https://trucesoftware.com*.

• **Learn to drive a manual transmission.** Driving "stick" can boost your attention while driving because you have to stay engaged with what you're doing to shift gears.

• **Stick to a strict "No Substance, No Sleepiness" driving policy.** Driving while sleepy or while using substances may be even riskier if you have ADHD. When in doubt, call an Uber or Lyft. It'll be worth avoiding a life-endangering mistake.

PART THREE

principles for living well with ADHD

In this part of the book, we'll widen our focus from coping with specific problems and using particular tools to reflecting on the ultimate purpose of coping with ADHD and the broad, big ideas that undergird this book's approach to living well.

26

what are your *whys*?

You *can* learn skills to better manage the impact of ADHD on your life. It's also true that learning these skills when you have ADHD will involve struggle, false starts, and coping with self-doubt. At those times, tapping into your big-picture motivation—your *whys*—can help you recommit to the process and keep moving forward.

> Your *whys* are your answers to the question
> "Why am I striving to learn skills to manage ADHD?"

Your *whys* also represent your vision for what living well with ADHD looks like for you. They're something you get to choose and something no one else can choose for you. What do you want your life to look like? Who do you want to be in the world? How do you want to show up for yourself and others? Without *whys* guiding your work, this book can read like a complex recipe for becoming the perfect worker or an overwhelming list of tasks that you're never going to complete. But with your *whys* leading the way, you will be able to choose the skills that will move you most in a meaningful direction.

To start contemplating your *whys*, write a bit in response to each prompt below.

What are the most important and meaningful areas of your life for living well? Your answers might include career, learning, family, friends, partner, health, leisure activities, volunteer work, spiritual community, engagement with nature, or other communities.

_____

_____

_____

_____

In which of these areas do you most wish to make positive changes right now?

_____

_____

_____

_____

If you could make a positive change in one of these areas, what would that look like?

_____

_____

_____

_____

Writing Your Whys

Remember, your *whys* are your answers to the question "Why am I striving to learn skills to manage ADHD?" Looking back at what you wrote and using the guidelines below, create the first draft of your *whys*.

- Phrase *why*s as what you want to **move toward** instead of what you want to avoid. For example:
  - ~~Avoid getting fired~~ To be a reliable and trustworthy team member to my coworkers
  - ~~Get my partner to stop nagging me~~ To be helpful to and mutually supportive of my partner
  - ~~To be less stressed out on a daily basis~~ To take good care of my mind and body.
- Phrase *why*s as something you can **continue** to move toward versus something you can check off a list.
  - ~~To get a high paying job~~ To earn enough money to support myself and ski as much as I can
  - ~~To get married~~ To sustain a long-term relationship with someone that's good for them and me
  - ~~To earn a PhD~~ To continue to challenge myself intellectually and contribute to my field

Here are some more examples:

- To show my kids that you can overcome challenges and not be perfect and still be a good dad
- To be a caring, supportive partner and a loving dog mom
- To be a trustworthy member of my church and a contributor to their charitable efforts
- To learn as much as I can throughout my life and use that learning to help others
- To cope with what life throws at me and connect with others

Your turn! Remember, phrase *why*s as something you can *keep moving toward*.

Why am I striving to learn skills to manage ADHD?

_____

_____

_____

Nice work! Remember, you can revise your *why*s whenever you want to. What is most meaningful can shift and change throughout your life. It's up to you.

What Next?

I recommend centering your *why*s when setting goals and deciding which skills you want to work on from this book. I also recommend you revisit your *why*s from time to time to refill your motivation and remind yourself of your purpose. Maybe even post your *why*s as a reminder in your home, workspace, or somewhere on your laptop or phone. (***Why*** not?)*

---

*I am very sorry. I couldn't resist.

27

the principles

I initially wanted to write this chapter first and to put it at the beginning of the book. As a professor by day, my inclination is to think in terms of big, abstract concepts and *then* to think about how those concepts apply in specific situations. But ultimately I'm glad I put this chapter last in the book and wrote it after writing about all the specific skills and examples that came before. Saving the Principles until the end allowed me to identify what is truly at the core of my approach to helping people with ADHD live better lives.*

Living well with ADHD is a matter of meeting each difficult moment with increasing levels of skill and self-acceptance. It would be impossible for me to write a book that could address every situation and challenge you will encounter as a person living with ADHD. And so there's value in naming and framing the core ideas that lie underneath the changes in thinking, feeling, and acting that can help you live better. Some of the Principles are about the way you think about or make meaning out of your experience with ADHD, and others are about how you respond through your actions. There are at least four ways you can use these Principles:

---

*Also, my book proposal originally included a possible 30-plus principles instead of the 14 I have here. You're welcome. ☺

1. To **adapt** the tools and strategies in this book to fit better with your own life

2. To **invent** totally new tools and strategies for living with ADHD

3. To help you **remember** to use the tools and strategies during crucial moments

4. To **replenish** your spirit when living with ADHD has left you feeling depleted

So even if you've decided to start your use of this book by reading this chapter, I invite you to come back and revisit it as you work through the specific recommendations in other sections.

You're Doing a Hard Thing

To live with ADHD is to face daily challenges. You didn't have a choice about having ADHD, but you have a choice in how you'll respond to the challenges it presents. But it isn't easy, and it's okay—even necessary—to acknowledge the moments when coping with ADHD is difficult. You're not deficient; you're experiencing challenges that some people will never experience. Be patient with yourself.

You're > ADHD

You could read this principle as "You're [more than] ADHD" or "You're [greater than] ADHD." I think they have slightly different meanings, and I mean both.

You're more than ADHD: Every person is more than a single adjective, label, or single fact about them. Living well with ADHD is just one aspect of you. You have important strengths, gifts, and talents. Living well is as much about cultivating and celebrating those talents as it is about managing ADHD. And you're greater than ADHD: You can move toward your goals and display your strengths, even while you cope with your symptoms.

This principle is also about deciding how you want to relate to ADHD in terms of your identity. Some people identify ADHD as the reason they have positive attributes like creativity or an outgoing nature. This is a valid choice, but it's not the only choice. It's also valid to see your positive attributes as something true of yourself, outside of your ADHD. And it's valid to be completely frustrated by ADHD and see it as something outside of your identity. Any of these ways of relating to your ADHD can be valid if it helps you to *live well*.

Center Your *Whys*

Your *whys* are what living well means to you. They're your North Star—what you want your life to be about and what you'll use when you're deciding what big goals to pursue. Your *whys* can become your motivation for learning how to better live with your ADHD. Notice: These are *your whys*, not the *whys* of your parents, your partner, your boss, or your fifth-grade teacher. If you're not sure what your *whys* are, that's a good place to start exploring. Use your *whys* to set your goals. Then your work to manage your ADHD will be *about* something more.

Find Your Niche

In the field of ecology, a niche is the set of conditions in which a plant or animal thrives best. People engage in *niche picking* (mentioned earlier) when they seek out places, people, and activities that work best with their abilities and interests. Finding your niche is about giving yourself permission to actively choose the settings and activities in which you can best thrive and live out your *whys*. It's about realizing that you may be unknowingly following rules that limit your choices and becoming more flexible in choosing the life that best fits your strengths.

Stay in Your Lane

This principle can sound limiting, but that's not how I mean it. By "stay in your lane,"* I mean going at your own pace toward your chosen goals without comparing yourself to other people. It means releasing yourself from self-judgment and comparison anxiety that doesn't serve you. Comparison is not only the thief of joy—it's a distraction that takes your eyes off what really matters.

Become a Tool Collector

The more tools you gather and skills you learn, the better you will be able to manage ADHD's many challenges toward a life well lived. This will be a lifelong journey, but one that you can view in terms of making progress and getting to know yourself better over time. Try to be open to as wide a variety of tools as possible, including medications, skills, professional assistance, and supportive relationships. The only way to know what works is to test it out. At the same time . . .

No One Thing Always Works

I said this at the beginning of the book, and I'll say it again: No tool is going to meet all the needs you have in terms of managing your ADHD. And it is damn hard to know in a given situation *which* tool is going to work. Life moves fast, and it's complicated. If something doesn't work in a particular moment, it doesn't mean that tool is useless, and it doesn't mean that you screwed up. You might need more practice to figure out exactly how to make a tool work for you. Or you may need a different strategy in that situation. Or you may never know why

---

*I can't remember where I first heard this idea, but it has been essential in raising an amazing child who is developing his skills at a different pace than his peers.

something didn't work that one time. It's frustrating, but it's just the way life is sometimes. Living well is about rolling with those moments, practicing self-compassion, and still trying again.

Failures Tell You What to Try Next

The idea "learn from your mistakes" seems beyond cliché. But when trying to build a toolbox and figure out what works, looking squarely at failures—times when the tools you tried to use didn't work—is essential to growing in *living well* with your ADHD. When something goes wrong, it can be painful to think through the process that led you to where you are. But if you can cultivate a grain of curiosity in the face of failure, you have the power to use what you learn to cope better next time. It can be exhausting, but you might just hit on a new way of making your life work.

Offload Self-Regulation

ADHD makes it harder for you to bring your behavior in line with your intentions and to guide your own behavior toward goals over time. Reduce the impact of ADHD on your life by creating situations that help you regulate and reduce the need to self-regulate. Create environments that prompt the actions you need to take. Boost motivation by setting up more frequent feedback and check-ins. Look for creative ways to hack your environment to support self-regulation.

Reflect on What's Going on Inside

Living well with ADHD is about understanding how it relates to what others can't see—your thoughts and feelings. Thoughts and feelings don't cause ADHD itself, but they play an important role in how you cope with it. What do you feel inside that you might be trying to escape from? What are you saying to yourself, and what stories are you telling yourself? These can all influence how you cope with ADHD in your life. And fortunately, these are also things you can change or learn to respond to differently.

Get Curious about How You Avoid

A lot of our daily behaviors happen on autopilot. We move through life automatically moving toward things that make us feel good, and—even more often—*we do things that let us escape* from what feels scary, uncomfortable, dull, or ugh. The symptoms of ADHD can make it even easier to do these automatic avoidance moves, but these can prevent you from really moving in the direction of your meaningful goals. As you consider what's going on inside, get extra-curious about what happens in the split seconds when you turn your mind away from what feels a little icky. Catching yourself in these moments can give you the chance to choose consciously.

Connect to Thrive

ADHD can make you feel separate from other people in ways that can be deeply painful. Yet a key move toward living well is cultivating supportive relationships with other people and tapping into the strength that comes from being vulnerable with others. "Finding your people" is a lifelong process, but it's a life-giving one as well.

Celebrate (Sm)All Wins

By this I mean celebrate **all** wins, even (and maybe especially) the small ones. People are distracted and wrapped up in their own lives and their own perspectives. They may not notice small but crucial moments of success in your movement toward living better with your ADHD. And you might not feel like small bits of progress are worthy of self-praise. But *you must notice and praise yourself for each positive step* if you want to progress! It's not a luxury—it's how behavior works. What is rewarded is repeated. Praise your own progress and that of others and the outcomes will follow.

Change Is Always Possible

This is not a platitude or a wish. It's a scientific fact based on everything we know about human behavior. It doesn't mean it's easy. It doesn't mean every *outcome* is possible. What it means is that, with the right understanding of your situation and your capabilities, and with the right support, you can always learn new skills and ways of living with your ADHD. And your belief in your capacity to change is, itself, an important step toward that change.

Your Principles for Living Well with ADHD

Please add the wisdom you've gained from your own experience about how to live well with ADHD. If you have a moment, please share them with me at *lknouse@richmond.edu*.

_____

_____

_____

resources

No matter how hard you work on your Toolbox, sometimes you need to call in an expert. Following are sources of outside support that can support living well with ADHD. This list refers frequently to *Taking Charge of Adult ADHD* (Russell A. Barkley, 2nd ed., The Guilford Press, 2022), which provides more comprehensive recommendations for several of these topics.

A Professional ADHD Evaluation

ADHD is among the most difficult mental health conditions to diagnose accurately for the following reasons:

- Many other mental health conditions can cause problems with distractibility and motivation, such as depression, anxiety disorders, and bipolar disorder.

- Many medical conditions or other lifestyle factors can cause ADHD-like symptoms such as thyroid problems, sleep apnea, and insomnia.

- ADHD often co-occurs with other mental health conditions, so clinicians must carefully tease these apart.

- ADHD is a developmental disorder, which means it affects people across their lifetime. A solid evaluation needs to collect information about your history and experiences earlier in life.

- It's recommended that evaluations include information not just from you, but from other people who know you well.

- A good evaluation will result in specific treatment recommendations tailored to your needs.

For all these reasons and more, you should seek out a thorough, professional ADHD evaluation if you have not already received one. ADHD is not a condition that can be diagnosed accurately in a 30- to 60-minute online assessment, and it's definitely not something you can diagnose with a questionnaire or online quiz. Even if you have had an evaluation earlier in life, an updated evaluation can help to reveal new potential ways of addressing your ADHD-related problems. You can find ADHD specialists using the lists provided by region at *https://chadd.org, https://apsard.org,* and *www.additudemag.com.* In Canada, try the *www.caddra.ca* website. In Europe, try the website for the European Network Adult ADHD (*www.eunetworkadultadhd.com*).

For in-depth information on how to get a good evaluation, see *Taking Charge of Adult ADHD* and read Step One: To Get Started, Get Evaluated.

Cognitive-Behavioral Therapy for ADHD

If you've found the vibe of this book interesting or helpful but are having trouble applying the tools in your daily life—which is understandable; changing your behavior is hard—then you might enjoy and benefit from working with a therapist trained in cognitive-behavioral therapy (CBT) for adult ADHD.

You may have heard of CBT before. CBT is really a family of treatment approaches, each one tailored for a particular problem like depression, obsessive-compulsive disorder, phobias, or bipolar disorder. Over the past 20 years or so, psychologists have developed a flavor of CBT specifically tailored to the needs of people with ADHD.

Most importantly, CBT approaches are frequently *tested in research studies to see if they actually work.* You can visit this website to view a list of research-supported psychotherapies, and you'll notice that many CBT approaches appear on the lists—including CBT for adult ADHD: *https://div12.org/treatments.*

The different flavors of CBT share the following features:

- CBT helps you learn skills to target specific problems and meet your goals.

- CBT is mostly about the here-and-now. You might discuss your past history and struggles to help you understand the present, but the focus will be on what you can do about your difficulties today.

- CBT helps you understand how your thoughts, emotions, and actions all influence each other and looks for ways to help you try out new ways of thinking and acting to get to your goals. As this book recommends, you'll be invited to try out different strategies in your real life.

- CBT tends to be more targeted and time limited than some other therapies. The aim is to help you reach your goals, so you can move forward with your new skills without needing to be in therapy your whole life (although you might drop back in from time to time for some support or skills coaching).

- In CBT your therapist will act as a partner and coach as you learn new things about yourself and as you try out new skills. It's not like going to the dentist. It's more like working with a personal trainer.

CBT for adult ADHD will specifically involve:

- Setting your personal goals for therapy related to the problems that you most want to resolve

- Education about the nature of ADHD and the rationale for treatment

- Exercises to help you understand how your thoughts, feelings, and behaviors related to ADHD all influence one another

- Structured sessions that involve identifying new skills like the ones in this book and then planning how you will practice them in daily life between sessions; when you return, you'll discuss how practice went and troubleshoot as you go

- Flexible support from your therapist to try new things and modify if things don't go as planned

How do you know if a therapist you might want to see practices CBT? It can be *very* hard to tell because there are no regulations on who can claim that they practice CBT, and unfortunately some studies have shown that therapists claiming to use CBT aren't really using the core elements that matter most.

First, check whether a therapist belongs to the Association for Behavioral and Cognitive Therapies, which is the premier professional organization for CBT therapists. You can search for a therapist in their online directory at *www.abct.org*. But just because someone isn't in that directory doesn't mean they might not be a stellar CBT therapist.

Second, you can use the list of CBT characteristics above to help you develop questions for a prospective therapist about their approach. You can also ask:

- Do you have specific training in CBT for adult ADHD, such as training during graduate school or attending workshops?
- Will you be using a therapist guide for CBT for adult ADHD that has been tested in research, such as those by Drs. Steven Safren, Mary Solanto, or J. Russell Ramsay?

Hopefully, if it seems right for you, this book has inspired you to be open to your own CBT journey!

Medication Treatment

For most adults with ADHD, medication treatment will be a crucial part of living well. If you've tried medications and decided they aren't for you, that's totally fine. But if you've tried medications and aren't satisfied with the effects or the side effects, if you've had difficulty communicating with your provider, or if you have the sense that you just aren't getting the maximum benefit from your medications, I encourage you to continue to demand better from your treatment. There are several varieties of ADHD medications as well as many different delivery systems, so trying just one drug type and delivery system (like Concerta or Focalin XR, which uses methylphenidate) and finding it inadequate does not mean that you will not do well on higher doses, on another drug type (amphetamines [Adderall XR, Vyvanse], anti-hypertensives [guanfacine or clonidine XR], norepinephrine reuptake inhibitors [Strattera, Qelbree], bupropion [Wellbutrin]) or using a different delivery system (pills, time release pellets, osmotic pump, skin patch, liquid time release, delayed onset taken the night before [Jornay PM]).

This book doesn't focus on medication, but I encourage you to check out Change Your Brain: Medications for Mastering ADHD in *Taking Charge of Adult ADHD* for comprehensive advice on understanding medication options and finding a provider.

Couples, Family, or Supportive Counseling

You might consider couples counseling or family therapy if there's a lot of conflict or instability in these relationships or if all members aren't getting what they need.

Make sure when looking for a couples or family therapist that you inform them about your ADHD and ask whether they have experience working with couples or families where ADHD is in the mix.

Some readers may benefit from therapy that's not specifically focused on skills for adult ADHD, but instead provides a place to get general support.

What's the difference between CBT for adult ADHD and supportive counseling? Imagine that you're a basketball player. CBT for adult ADHD is sort of like going to practice for basketball—where you focus on honing specific skills—while supportive counseling is more like the workouts you do in the gym to keep up your general fitness level. Both are potentially useful, but one is more focused on a specific set of skills.

Still, it's probably a good idea to ask whether your supportive counselor or therapist has experience working with adults with ADHD before you decide to commit.

ADHD Coaching

Life coaching for people with ADHD seems to be on the rise, but it can be hard to understand the difference between coaching and therapy. Coaching can be useful for people with ADHD, and there are undoubtedly many caring and skilled coaches, but it's important to understand what coaching is and isn't so that you can make an informed decision.

- The purpose of coaching is to help people work through specific problems, but not necessarily to help them develop skills that will last beyond the coaching relationship.

- Coaches are not psychologists, social workers, or counselors and don't claim to be. They're not required to have training in treating any mental health condition, so coaching isn't a substitute for ADHD treatment. It also isn't usually covered by health insurance.

- The practice of coaching isn't regulated by the government. Unlike health professionals, there is no state licensing process for coaches. Coaches may earn certifications from national coaching organizations, and these can be a mark of the quality of the coach, but basically anyone can claim to be an ADHD coach.

If you're considering working with an ADHD coach, consider asking the following:

- What training have you completed in coaching? Have you completed any education or training specific to ADHD?

- Do you hold any certifications from national coaching organizations for ADHD coaches?

- What will be the goals of our work together, and how will we know that coaching is complete?

- How will our work fit in with my other ADHD treatments?

index

Note. *n* following a page number indicates a note.

Absorbing information, 116–123, 153. *See also* Information
Academic paths, 85–88, 167–178
Acceptance, 63
Accommodations, 172–175
Accountability groups, 34. *See also* Accountability Partners
Accountability Partners. *See also* Relationships; Support from others
  completing tasks accurately and, 87
  eating well and, 181
  getting started and restarted and, 93–94, 95
  making thoughtful decisions and, 144, 147
  managing money and, 192
  managing strong emotions and, 136
  overview, 33–36
  planning and prioritizing and, 84
  sticking with and finishing a task and, 98, 99
Action-oriented approach, 1–2
Active listening, 122. *See also* Listening to others
ADHD coaching. *See* Coaching
ADHD overview, vii–viii, 1–3
ADHD Toolbox. *See also* Menu of moves; *individual devices; individual skills; individual strategies*
  collecting tools, skills, and strategies, 204
  keeping an open mind about, 12–13
  overview, vii–viii, 7, 8–9, 11–13, 55
  principles for living well and, 202
  tools in, 12–13

Alarms
  building tidying rituals/habits and, 165
  eating well and, 181
  making thoughtful decisions and, 144
  managing money and, 192
  overview, 23–24
  showing up on time and, 60
  switching gears when necessary, 107
Alcohol use, 185–186
All-or-nothing thinking, 100–102
Americans with Disabilities Act (ADA), 172–173
Anger, 130–139. *See also* Emotions
Anxiety, 6, 94, 101
Apologies. *See also* Effective Apologies
  forgetting and, 70
  getting started and restarted and, 95
  keeping commitments to others and, 115
  making thoughtful decisions and, 148
  managing strong emotions and, 139
  overview, 50–52, 53
  reducing the impact of ADHD on relationships and, 157
Appointments. *See also* Scheduling; Time organization
  forgetting and, 67–68, 76
  keeping commitments to others and, 110–115
Appreciation, 63, 155–156
Apps. *See* Smartphone use; Technology
Asking for what you want, 49–50
Assessment, 6, 209–210
Assignments, 85–88

215

about the authors

Laura E. Knouse, PhD, is Professor of Psychology at the University of Richmond. She is an expert in studying and treating ADHD in adults. Her research focuses on the skills people need to cope with ADHD symptoms and achieve their goals—and the most effective ways to teach them. Dr. Knouse lives in Richmond, Virginia, with her husband and two children.

Russell A. Barkley, PhD, ABPP, ABCN, before retiring in 2021, served on the faculties of the University of Massachusetts Medical Center, the Medical University of South Carolina, and Virginia Commonwealth University. Dr. Barkley is the author of numerous books, six assessment scales, and more than 300 scientific articles and book chapters on ADHD and related disorders. He is the recipient of awards from the American Academy of Pediatrics and the American Psychological Association, among other honors. His website is *www.russellbarkley.org*.